When Painkillers Become Dangerous

When
Painkillers
Become
Dangerous

What Everyone Needs to Know about
OxyContin and Other Prescription Drugs

DREW PINSKY, M.D.

Marvin D. Seppala, M.D.

Robert J. Meyers, Ph.D.

John Gardin, Ph.D.

William White, M.A.

Stephanie Brown, Ph.D.

HAZELDEN

Hazelden, Center City, Minnesota 55012-0176

1-800-328-0094   1-651-213-4590 (Fax)   www.hazelden.org

ISBN-13: 978-1-59285-107-2

Library of Congress Cataloging-in-Publication Data

When painkillers become dangerous : what everyone needs to know about Oxycontin
and other prescription drugs / Drew Pinsky ... [et al.].
     p. cm.
  Includes bibliographical references and index.
  ISBN 1-59285-107-X
    1. Narcotic habit—Popular works. 2. Analgesics—Popular works. 3. Sedatives—
  Popular works. 4. Oxycodone—Popular works. I. Pinsky, Drew.

RC566.W48 2004
616.86'06—dc22

                                                                    2004052261

Editor's note
Some of the stories found in this book are composites of actual situations. Other stories found in this book were created by the authors to represent the common experiences of individuals and their families who have dealt with addiction to prescription medication. Any resemblance to a specific person, living or dead, or to a specific event is coincidental.

This book is not intended as a substitute for the medical advice of physicians. The reader should consult a physician in matters relating to his or her health.

The following brand names appear in this book: CYLERT, DESOXYN, DILAUDID, LUMINAL, NEMBUTAL, and PLACIDYL are registered trademarks of Abbott Laboratories; ANTABUSE, ATIVAN, and EQUANIL are registered trademarks of American Home Products Corporation; VICOPROFEN is a registered trademark of BASF K & F; MILTOWN is a registered trademark of Carter-Wallace, Inc.; PERCOCET is a registered trademark of DuPont Merck Pharmaceutical Company; SECONAL and TUINAL are registered trademarks of Eli Lilly and Company; PERCODAN is a registered trademark of Endo Pharmaceuticals Inc.; KLONOPIN is a registered trademark of Hoffmann-La Roche Inc.; LIBRIUM is a registered trademark of ICN Pharmaceuticals, Inc.; SUBLIMAZE is a registered trademark of Johnson & Johnson; VICODIN is a registered trademark of Knoll Pharmaceutical Company; RITALIN is a registered trademark of Novartis Corporation; XANAX is a registered trademark of Pharmacia & Upjohn Company; OXYCONTIN is a registered trademark of Purdue Pharma L.P.; AMYTAL is a registered trademark of Ranbaxy Pharmaceuticals Inc.; VALIUM is a registered trademark of Roche Products Inc.; DEMEROL is a registered trademark of Sanofi-Synthelabo Inc.; DEXEDRINE is a registered trademark of Smithkline Beckman Corporation; TALWIN is a registered trademark of Sterling Drug Inc.; LORTAB is a registered trademark of UCB Phip, Inc.; MARINOL is a registered trademark of Unimed Pharmaceuticals, Inc.; LORTAB ASA is a registered trademark of Whitby Pharmaceuticals, Inc.

2018   8 7 6

Cover design by David Spohn
Interior design and typesetting by Kinne Design

IF SOME NEW AND TERRIBLE DISEASE were suddenly to strike us here in America—a disease of unknown cause, possibly due to noxious gas or poison in our soil, air, or water, it would be treated as a national emergency, with our whole citizenry uniting as a man to fight it.

Let us suppose the disease to have so harmful an effect on the nervous system that [millions of] people in our country would go insane for periods lasting from a few hours to weeks or months and recurring repetitively. . . .

Let us further suppose that during these spells of insanity, acts of so destructive a nature would be committed that the material and spiritual lives of whole families would be in jeopardy. . . . Work in business, industry, professions and factories would be crippled, sabotaged or left undone. . . .

Finally, let us imagine this poison or disease to have the peculiar property of so altering a person's judgment, so brainwashing him, that he would be unable to see that he had become ill at all; actually so perverting and so distorting his view of life that he would wish with all his might to go on being ill.

The dread disease envisioned above is actually here. It is alcoholism.

— *THE ROUNDABOUT*

— *Ruth Fox, M.D.*
Medical Advisor
National Council on Alcoholism

From Ruth Fox, "Imagine Such a Disease . . . ," reprinted from *AA Grapevine* 23, no. 9 (February 1967): 23.

Contents

OxyContin and Other Prescription Pain Medication, 1
HOW ADDICTION DEVELOPS
Drew Pinsky, M.D.

How Addiction Treatment Works, 31
Marvin D. Seppala, M.D.

How to Intervene on a Loved One's Addiction, 65
Robert J. Meyers, Ph.D., and John Gardin, Ph.D.

OxyContin Addiction, 99
A NEW DRUG, BUT AN OLD PROBLEM
William White, M.A.

Addiction As a Family Disease, 139
Stephanie Brown, Ph.D.

OxyContin and Other Prescription Pain Medication

HOW ADDICTION DEVELOPS

Drew Pinsky, M.D.

"Get in there and push six milligrams of morphine on that post-op femur. And debride his heel while you're in there." The orthopedic resident glared down at me with disdain. "Get on it."

I, a wide-eyed third-year med student, ran into the open ward with six beds arrayed about the periphery of the dormitory. I found Mr. Resnick writhing in pain. He was too distressed to notice my presence. I grabbed his IV tubing, kinked off above the port, and slowly injected the morphine. Within seconds, his breathing became slower and deeper. A calmness swept across his face. As he became more comfortable, I remember my sense of awe and excitement that I had been able to help this man who had been suffering.

This was my first experience as a medical student administering an opiate to a patient. I cannot express to you my satisfaction at having been able to help this man so vividly and quickly. After all, this is what those of us who enter helping professions expect and hope from our careers; and rarely do we get to experience this sense of triumph so thoroughly as with our ability to take away pain. Every physician learns early that we can reliably and easily relieve pain with opiates.

Mr. Resnick had been in a motorcycle accident and suffered multiple injuries. He was an addict, but at that point in my training, I did not understand what that meant. It seemed to me that he was frequently demanding pain medication. But why not? He had just had an operation on his leg. The more he demanded, the more I dutifully came running with the morphine.

As time went along, Mr. Resnick told me about his addiction to heroin. I was shocked. He was a college graduate. He maintained a small business. Heroin? How could that be? When it came time for discharge, I made sure that he had an adequate supply of Vicodin. He was extremely preoccupied with being certain of the amount and number of refills. I didn't think much of it at the time, and I agreed with him that he just needed to get out of the neighborhood where he lived and stay away from his heroin-using friends.

It sounds ridiculous in retrospect, but my lack of understanding of the disease of addiction probably did this man considerable harm. Was it wrong to give him opiates for his pain? No. He needed pain medication, and, in fact, because of his addiction and tolerance to opiates, he needed more than the average patient to control his pain. However, I had absolutely no understanding of the addictive disease process and how I might be contributing to it.

Addictive Diseases

I, like every medical student of my time, had essentially no training in addictive diseases. I was focused only on treating Mr. Resnick's orthopedic problems. He needed pain relief, and it never occurred to me to consider anything beyond that. If he had a drug problem, well certainly he had now learned his lesson, and no doubt, he would avoid all those bad influences that "made" him use drugs.

As a doctor, I felt triumphant in my ability to help this man and rescue him from his suffering. Given what had happened to him as a result of his drug use, I couldn't imagine he would continue using. If he did continue, well, he just needed to take my direction more seriously. If he still continued to use drugs, well, then that was his problem.

Mr. Resnick's case highlights the complications of using medication to alleviate human suffering when the caregiver does not have a sophisticated understanding of addiction. This patient needed pain medication, and he needed specific referrals and treatment for the disease—addiction—that put him at risk for the motorcycle accident in the first place. Mr. Resnick's addiction became even more difficult to treat because of the complexity of trying to manage his pain with the very chemicals to which he was addicted. Later in this chapter, you will see how heroin, morphine, and Vicodin are related substances.

These complex issues are becoming more prevalent every day. The statistics are alarming. The National Institute on Drug Abuse (NIDA) reports that in 1999 an estimated 4 million people (about 2 percent of the American population age twelve and older) were currently (in the previous month) using prescription drugs non-medically. Of these 4 million people, 2.6 million were misusing pain relievers, 1.3 million were misusing sedatives and tranquilizers, and 0.9 million were misusing stimulants.[1] These numbers obviously do not reflect the many thousands of people who may not recognize that they are misusing prescription medication but have become addicted as the result of following a doctor's orders.

NIDA further reports from its 2003 Monitoring the Future survey of eighth, tenth, and twelfth graders that 10.5 percent of twelfth graders report using Vicodin for non-medical purposes and 4.5 percent had used OxyContin without a prescription.[2]

We present in these pages a thorough examination of a growing problem for our country: addiction to prescription pain medication. We felt it was important to create a single, complete resource addressing this problem. Our focus will be on a specific drug in this class of medication: OxyContin. Throughout this book, we will look at the nature of addiction, its effect on the family, treatment modalities, and an intervention option.

How Pain Medication Works

Prescription pain medications are essentially all related by their common effect on the body's endorphin system. The molecules of the medication mimic the effects of the body's own endorphins, but are much more powerful and last for longer periods of time.

Endorphins are involved in many biological actions, including respiration, nausea, vomiting, pain modulation, and hormonal regulation. There are several types of endorphin receptors, including the delta, mu, and kappa receptors. Each of these three receptors is involved in different physiologic functions. The blocking of pain comes primarily from effects on the mu receptor. The emotional effects of pain medication are quite complex. Pain medications exert their effects on the limbic system, or what is considered the emotion center of the brain, and can in many individuals induce a sense of euphoria.

The Juice of the Poppy

Pain medications share a common historical heritage. Derivatives of the poppy flower, first cultivated around 3,400 B.C., have been used by humans for thousands of years. The term *opiate* describes naturally occurring and synthetic compounds directly derived from the poppy. The word *opioid* is used to describe any derivative of the opiate class. Opium contains a complex mix of sugars, proteins, fats, water, latex, gums, ammonia, sulphuric and lactic acids, and numerous alkaloids, most notably morphine, codeine, noscapine, papaverine, and thebaine. Although thebaine has no pain-relieving effect, it is used to synthesize other opioids which have become very popular: hydrocodone (Vicodin), hydromorphone (Dilaudid), and oxycodone (Percocet). OxyContin is a controlled release, high-concentration formulation of oxycodone.

The writings of Theophrastus (third century B.C.) are the first known reference to opium. The word *opium* derives from the Greek word for "juice of a plant." Opium was actually prepared from the juice of the poppy. The juice is derived from the seedpods of the flower. Ancient Sumerians, Assyrians, Babylonians, and Egyptians learned that smoking the extract causes pleasurable effects. Use of the plant later spread to Arabia, India, and China. In Europe, it was introduced by Paracelsus (1493–1541).

In the eighteenth century, opium smoking was popular in the Far East, and the opium trade was a very important source of income for the colonial rulers from England, Holland, and Spain. Opium contains a considerable number of different substances, and in the nineteenth century, these were isolated. Friedrich Sertürner was the first to extract one of these substances in its pure form. He called this chemical *morphine* after Morpheus, the Greek god of sleep or dreams.

People soon realized that morphine was indeed addictive, and they began looking for a non-addictive alternative—a fruitless search that continues until this day. There will never be a non-addictive opiate. In 1874, the English pharmacist C. R. Alder Wright boiled morphine and acetic acid to produce diacetylmorphine. This new compound was soon synthesized and put on the market under the brand name Heroin. Heroin was initially sold as a cough suppressant and quickly became popular. It was sold worldwide until it became very obvious that people were overusing this product. Distribution stopped in 1913. In chapter 4, William White presents a fascinating look at how pain remedies have been abused through the centuries. You will see that the human quest for pain relief has been a longstanding search.

History of OxyContin

Oxycodone was developed in Germany in the early years of the twentieth century. It has been available in Europe by injection and orally since 1917. Oral formulations were available in America in the 1950s, typically combined with another agent such as aspirin (Percodan) or acetaminophen (Percocet). These medications were taken orally, readily absorbed, and rapid acting, but they had a short duration of action and they were only available in low-dose formulations. Patients needed to take multiple pills at frequent intervals.

To solve this problem, OxyContin was developed as a twelve-hour slow-release medication to manage severe pain. OxyContin was quickly hailed as superior to morphine in terms of the lower incidence of side effects such as nausea or hallucinations. Doctors were able to maintain steady levels of pain medication in their patients, thereby increasing the pain-relief effects. OxyContin pills have a very high level of active opioid, which is enclosed in a wax matrix or capsule; this capsule is designed to release the opioid slowly. However, if one simply chews or crushes the pills, all of the oxycodone is released at once. Before long, people figured this out and OxyContin rapidly became a popular drug of abuse.

OxyContin is as much as twenty-five times stronger than a simple oxycodone tablet. The dose in a single OxyContin tablet is potentially dangerous but generally thought not to be of a high enough concentration to cause a person to stop breathing. However, when used with a central nervous system suppressant such as alcohol or a benzodiazepine like Xanax or Klonopin, the risk of death becomes very real. Most Oxy-Contin deaths arise from this phenomenon.

Addicts generally crush the pill and snort the drug, causing rapid absorption of large concentrations of oxycodone. The drug can also be injected but requires some preparation for this route of administration.

Addicts obtain OxyContin by purchasing it on the street or from Internet sites. Another common practice is visiting multiple physicians with well-rehearsed complaints that will compel a physician to prescribe OxyContin. There are also unscrupulous physicians who will write prescriptions for a fictitious patient to be filled by a pharmacist who may or may not explicitly collude with the physician. The tremendous increase in the use of pain medication in recent decades has added to the ease of availability. And, as you will come to see, the differences among medical specialties and the complexities of managing pain further add to the problem.

Sorting through the Hype

"Oxy" has entered the common lexicon of American adolescents. The media has been particularly enamored with stories about

OxyContin. They frequently portray the drug as heroin-like and unbelievably addicting. Catchy terminology like "hillbilly heroin" has entered the public consciousness. The media looks for the most sensational stories, giving the public the sense that OxyContin is more serious and dangerous than other types of addictive substances. Unfortunately, these news stories underplay the potential beneficial uses of OxyContin.

The fact is, the non-medical use of all prescription pain medication increased throughout the 1990s. While OxyContin is contributing to this rise, on a percentage basis, its contribution is not significant. The National Household Survey on Drug Abuse conducted by the Substance Abuse and Mental Health Services Administration (SAMHSA) revealed that between 2000 and 2001 the number of people who had used OxyContin non-medically once in their lifetime increased from 399,000 to 957,000, while the number of people who had used Vicodin non-medically increased from 6.7 million to 9.5 million.[3]

OxyContin prescriptions rose markedly soon after the drug was introduced—from 300,000 in 1996 to 6.8 million in 2001. It is important to note, however, that the number of prescriptions for other pain medications rose from 155 million in 1996 to 190 million in 2000.[4] While OxyContin is worth our attention and scrutiny, the fact is that it has become emblematic for a larger problem: the inappropriate use of all prescription pain medications.

What Is Addiction?

Addiction, as compared to abuse, is a biological disorder with a genetic basis whereby the motivational priorities of the mind become permanently altered. Abuse is any inappropriate or non-medical use of a substance, and as I pointed out, the abuse of opioids is quite common today. When opioids are abused with other central nervous system suppressants, the results can be very dangerous. People who abuse substances—as opposed to people who are addicted—can be influenced by persuasion and reason to stop abusing the substance. For instance, it has been repeatedly shown that the probability of a young person abusing a substance is inversely proportional to the perceived harm potentially caused by that substance.

Another way of saying this is that young people are less likely to abuse substances that they believe will harm them. On the other hand, this potential for harm has no influence once someone becomes addicted. An addict will no longer respond to reason or persuasion.

For some, the tasks of recovery from addiction are insurmountable. The drives of addiction are overwhelming, and if pain is a confounding factor, the possibility of abstinence and the colossal tasks of recovery are simply too much. Some patients elect to take the road of harm avoidance through what is called maintenance therapy, such as a methadone program (see pages 15–16). But the possibility of emotional change necessary for recovery is closed to these patients. The replacement drug, such as methadone, blocks many of the brain mechanisms that must be set in motion for emotional growth and the development of recovery. These patients are committed to a chronic state of affairs. Though harm avoidance may be lifesaving for some patients, abstinence-based recovery offers a richer alternative.

Genetics and Trauma

Addiction is a genetic disorder, which means addiction can be passed down to subsequent generations. Simply put, people from addicted or alcoholic families are predisposed—or at risk—to develop addiction themselves. Why, then, would such a predisposed individual ever touch drugs in the first place? The answer to this question depends on the psychobiology of the individual who seems to be looking for solutions to his or her emotional problems through drugs and alcohol.

In my experience, addicts who require inpatient treatment for their disease have experienced trauma as a common feature of their childhoods. For that group of patients, opiates or opioids hold a particular allure. By *trauma,* I am referring to interpersonal trauma, explicitly the experience of being powerless at the hands of parents or caregivers who were responsible for the safety and nurturance of these patients as children. Interpersonal trauma in early life is thought to be different than experiencing a natural disaster or living in a war-torn country. The two most common forms of interpersonal trauma are abuse and neglect.

Trauma is a common historical feature of the childhood of addicts. The fact that addiction is an inherited disease increases the likelihood that a person with addiction had a parent affected by the disease. This, in and of itself, is a source of trauma. An intoxicated parent is an abandoning parent. Trying to negotiate oneself in an alcoholic or addicted family can be traumatizing, and frequently, far more serious issues, such as abuse, emerge.

Neurobiological sciences are slowly developing a picture as to why trauma would set up someone for addiction. In the following pages, I will talk about the complex relationship between emotional development and brain function. The concepts I will discuss are based on the work of Allan N. Schore. Three of his books are cited in my notes if you are interested in doing further reading.[5]

Evidence of the effects of opiates on the brain's cingulate gyrus is slowly emerging. There is evidence that trauma survivors have abnormalities of the cingulate, particularly in the anterior region. Opiates may exploit these deficiencies. The cingulate is a region of the brain that developed as mammals evolved a need for longer periods of maternal nurturance. It is a part of the brain involved in our ability to screen or modulate pain, and it is probably involved in our capacity to feel nurtured. The effects on emotions involved in bonding and nurturance can be profound when the opiates are removed. Opiate withdrawal can literally feel like the grief of losing a loved one.

Furthermore, trauma survivors have tremendous difficulty regulating the intensity and duration of feelings, particularly negative feelings. Clinicians call these emotional reactions *deficiencies of affect regulation*. Children who experience trauma can grow into adults who lack strong internal coping systems. As adults, they feel inadequate and overwhelmed. They may unconsciously conclude that they didn't get what they needed while growing up so perhaps they are less worthy than others. One of the startling truths about these human beings is that experiences during early development, when the brain is forming new connections most rapidly, have a disproportionate influence on all else that is to follow.

Trauma results in deep feelings of lack of safety and security, and most tragically, it ruptures the relationship with and trust in one's primary caregivers. As a result of this rupture, a child loses his or her access to the primary means whereby we come to know ourselves. It is, in fact, through our relationship with our primary caregivers that we come to know and understand ourselves and others. We learn to identify feelings and understand intentionality. By seeing our feelings reflected in the faces of our caregivers, we move from merely being awash in emotions to being able to identify, understand, and regulate feeling states.

These primarily right brain activities allow for the development of the executive system called the orbiofrontal region of the brain. This structure sits at the intersection of the limbic (emotional), frontal (rational), and autonomic (visceral) regions of the brain. The regulation and integration of these systems develop as the result of mutual exchanges with our caregivers. Therefore, we naturally need to trust that we will not discover something terrifying or overwhelming in the process.

Trauma ruptures this trust. A child who is exposed to trauma discovers an overwhelming reality: The caregiver whom the child loves most does not see him or her as a separate feeling entity, rather, the caregiver sees him or her as an entity that can be easily exploited. Worse yet, the child might find in the caregiver the intention to inflict pain on him or her.

This type of relationship interferes with the child's alliance with the caregiver and aborts the child's normal process of emotional development. The child stops looking to the caregiver for nurturing feedback or validation of his or her feelings. The child's emotional growth stops at that stage and becomes reliant on more primitive means of affect regulation. A child can't continue along the developmental path of increasing complexity and integration of feelings without the ongoing emotional guidance of safe caregivers.

Lingering Effects of Trauma

Patients will often say to me that they have dealt with their traumatic pasts. They believe that they have effectively and willfully put the memories out of their minds. What they don't realize is that the remnant effects of past trauma on their brain function, on implicit procedural memory, impair their ability to work through emotions. The trauma of the past has left them with an inability to fully process these past events. So it is not merely depression, anxiety, or other psychiatric symptoms that fuel the pursuit of drugs. I think it is more accurate to consider the initial choice to use drugs as a bid for affect regulation, or as an attempt to find a solution to unmanageable feelings.

Symptoms that trauma survivors experience may include depression or anxiety but that does not seem to be sufficient to trigger the disease of addiction. Rather, patients seem to have fundamental deficiency of self; that is, they feel like they are less than others, worthless, and unable to manage their emotions. Not everyone with psychiatric symptoms uses drugs and alcohol to medicate their symptoms. Opiates and opioids are effective, at least superficially, at rescuing patients from the pain of a traumatic past. Many of my patients will report that, upon using an opiate or opioid, they felt okay for the first time—they felt "normal." From the first use, this becomes a compelling drive to use drugs.

Yet this is still not sufficient for the disease to develop. Addiction requires the activation of a genetically based bio-logical process where drugs continue to be pursued, even when they are no longer effective at helping the patient feel better. The drugs or alcohol are no longer working, yet the individual cannot stop the use. Biological drives and motiva-tional priorities have been set in motion that overwhelm the patient's use of higher brain functions such as judgment or decision-making.

More severe forms of trauma may result in a phenomenon called dissociation. A traumatized individual will actually disconnect from the overwhelming feelings associated with the trauma. How this occurs is now well understood. It is the result of a part of the nervous system called the autonomic system. This is made up of two opposing mechanisms: (1) the sympathetic, which causes the fight-or-flight response and

(2) the parasympathetic, which is the brakes or the inhibitory mechanism. In the face of interpersonal trauma, an individual switches from a state of hyper excitation (fight or flight) to a state of hyper inhibition when it is clear that there is no escape. Hyper inhibition is controlled by the main outflow of the parasympathetic system. Dissociation is a parasympathetic mechanism that is a remnant of death-feigning behaviors seen in less-evolved animals.

Dissociation may be a means of natural survival when a person is faced with an overwhelming threat. The problem arises when the traumatized person tends to rely on this primitive means of coping because trauma has short-circuited the potential for integration of these mechanisms with higher centers of the brain. This means the person begins to use dissociation across a broad range of stressors, particularly interpersonal conflicts. In states of dissociation, rage often emerges. And using drugs and alcohol can become a way to manage these overwhelming feelings.

Some children who have been physically or sexually abused actually learn to dissociate from their bodies. The child's body is the source of the chaotic and overwhelming stimuli shattering the child's ability to manage the experience. Using the only means he or she has to adapt and survive, the child learns to disconnect from the stimuli.

Because the dissociation results in the "parceling off" of bodily input from higher centers in the brain, pain may be the only means by which the traumatized individual can communicate his or her experiences of distress. The connections are not there to integrate the body with consciousness. Chronic pain patients who are addicted to opiates or opioids have a high incidence of physical and sexual abuse.[6] This suggests that the pain they experience may have a complex neuropsychological origin.

The Nature of Pain

The very nature of pain is most elusive. Pain refers to an event in the brain registered as an unpleasant experience, but what exactly that is and how it occurs is exceedingly complex. Even the world's experts cannot reach a consensus. In 1986, the International Association for the Study of Pain defined pain as "an unpleasant sensory and motional experience associated with actual or potential tissue damage or described in terms of such damage."[7]

Pain under normal circumstances is a terrifically complex process. Sensors in the skin and soft tissue send messages to the spinal cord via peripheral nerves. Processing occurs in the spinal cord, which then sends messages to the brain. There is well-documented evidence that injury at almost any step along this journey can result in chronic physiological changes that are then experienced as chronic pain.[8]

So how should pain be treated in patients, particularly if they have a biological genetic predisposition for addiction? Most pain experts would be inclined to advocate an approach called "rational polypharmacy." Usually this includes the use of opiates or opioids if the goal is complete pain control. It is not uncommon to see a pain patient on eight or nine different medications in an attempt to attack the pain by means of multiple mechanisms. Little regard is given to assessing the patient for the potential of addiction. The goal is pain control.

Some caregivers, even within the field of addiction medicine, are increasingly advocating a similar approach for patients with a previous addiction. This would fall under the umbrella of what has come to be called *harm avoidance*. The harm avoidance approach asserts that a disease has been activated with a very poor prognosis: opiate addiction. Because the brain chemistry has been permanently altered, the goal will not be remission of the disease process. Rather, it will be the avoidance of the harm that comes from the ongoing pursuit of opiates.

Pain itself can be a source of harm and a reason for pursuing the opiate. Uncontrolled pain has been clearly shown to be destructive to patients' lives. The pain control is generally accomplished by providing the patient with increasing doses of long-acting opioids, like methadone, and preventing withdrawal and the preoccupation with procuring the drugs.

Methadone, however, commits a patient to chronic illness. Harm avoidance, or maintenance therapy, is being increasingly urged as the intervention of choice even when pain is not a prominent issue in a patient's addiction. It is a viable alternative in some cases, but not if one intends to return to a high level of functioning in life. I would remind readers that while harm avoidance is offered as a treatment strategy for some patients, it is considered out of the question for professionals such as doctors, nurses, or airline pilots who must return to their work unimpaired. I believe a more sophisticated approach is an attempt to induce remission through the recovery process.

Further complicating matters is the observation that opiates themselves may perpetuate pain by lowering the thresholds for pain tolerance. Chronic use of opiates is also thought to cause a syndrome of recurrent low-grade withdrawal. As the opiate wears off, the individual begins experiencing symptoms of withdrawal (such as deep despair and back and leg pain), urging the patient on to his or her next dose of opiate.

A Physician's Dilemma

Many patients begin opiate use in an attempt to control a common symptom: back pain. They are never told, oftentimes, that opiates perpetuate the symptom for which they are taking the medication in the first place. This is not to say that every opiate user with back pain must immediately stop their medication. I can, however, share with you that I have never admitted a patient to my chemical dependency unit for whom pain, wherever it was localized, did not improve markedly with discontinuing opiates. The brain will go to great lengths to get the drug to which it has become addicted. This includes distorting the individual's feelings and thought processes and, many times, causing pain. And as we have discussed, trauma further complicates the picture.

Most people who become addicted to prescription pain medication do not set out with any goal other than to control pain. And certainly it is generally not the physician's intent to harm a patient by colluding in the evolution of addiction. Although there are those physicians who will provide patients with medication for whatever the patient's whim dictates, these doctors tend to be motivated by money or may be addicts themselves. Recklessness arises from their denial of their own disease. These physicians feel justified in providing patients with medication, and they deny the potential for negative effects, which they refuse to see in their own use. Most physicians, however, merely unintentionally fumble into trouble with a patient, much like my own story with Mr. Resnick, because of well-meaning attempts to care for a patient.

Unfortunately, when the addiction is triggered and the patient returns to a doctor with increasing complaints and demands for more medication, doctors tend to make this the patient's problem. The physician perceives the patient as demanding and difficult, rather than recognizing that the patient has a new or reactivated condition that needs assessment, referral, and treatment.

Physicians are often reluctant to address these issues with the patient because the patient may perceive the doctor as moralizing or judgmental by suggesting a diagnosis of addiction. Physicians are also uncomfortable with the stigma associated with addiction. They fear that the patient will be outraged by this diagnosis, an experience all too often encountered by physicians.

Since denial is a defining feature of addiction, even when the addiction has been accidentally triggered through appropriate medical management, a patient will fight fiercely against the suggestion that he or she is an addict. Denial fuels righteous indignation: "What do you mean? I just want my pain controlled." More often than not, neither the patient nor the physician understands the difficulty of coming to terms with the opiate's addictive effect on the brain.

Finally, what about patients, such as those suffering from cancer, with pain at the end of their lives? These are the patients for whom drugs like OxyContin were created. Opiates and opioids are universally hailed as the standards for reducing human suffering in these desperate situations. Whatever the patient needs to be comfortable is generally the guiding principle. OxyContin has been an extremely important addition to the arsenal of the treatment of pain in this setting.

Yet, even here, there can be controversy. Doctors get so many mixed messages about the use of pain medication that they may be reluctant to use them when they are universally accepted as absolutely appropriate and necessary.[9] Dr. Richard Brown of the University of Wisconsin School of Medicine has discovered in his research that physicians sometimes do not prescribe enough pain medication. He gave a group of physicians a set of hypothetical patients and compared their use of pain medications with that proposed for the same hypothetical patients by a group of experts. Brown found that compared to the experts, the two thousand physicians who participated in the study were reluctant to prescribe opiates. Five percent underprescribed medication for severe cancer pain—a decision that can cause great suffering for a patient.

Addiction Solutions

In chapter 2, Dr. Marvin D. Seppala specifically addresses the issues commonly encountered by the prescription medication addict. You'll also learn about how Twelve Step recovery works. The Twelve Step model for treatment is a time-honored approach, which serves as the foundation in most treatment facilities, and it is effective for the prescription pain medication addict.

First of all, the Twelve Step model emphasizes fellowship. Addicts, and especially trauma survivors, have difficulty opening up emotionally if they do not feel that they are going to be completely understood. The Twelve Step fellowship provides them with a community where they can feel completely understood.

Equally as important, addicts have a keen sense of when another addict has not fully embraced the process of treatment. They know when the disease is continuing to hold the patient in the grip of distorted priorities. They know it in themselves, and they have experience seeing it in their peers. And they do not hesitate to confront the disease.

One of the first priorities in recovery is to re-establish connection with others so that the addict may regain access to the normal developmental mechanisms. This will allow the person to continue along the path of developing more complex and integrated means of regulating feelings. This begins by exploring the feelings associated with being powerless over this condition we call addiction.

Remember, powerlessness is a terribly painful issue for

the trauma survivor. Having been exposed to trauma, he or she becomes hypervigilant and even on guard against circumstances or relationships that could leave him or her feeling powerless. In order to get past these feelings, an addict in early recovery has to be willing to trust the availability of another person. We call that person a *sponsor* in the Twelve Step program.

Beyond Powerlessness

Merely identifying and experiencing powerlessness is usually not enough to get patients to let go of the grandiose need to control their environment. In order to let go and believe that they will not be exploited or abused, they must be willing to have faith—faith that if they let go, things will still turn out all right. This is where the Higher Power concept becomes important to patients' recovery. Patients will often describe this experience as the most important in the process of recovery.

The Twelve Step process re-establishes trust and connection with caring others. Increasingly intense emotional experiences are encouraged as the Steps progress.

Typically, feelings of shame and guilt are explored in the Fourth and Fifth Steps. These feelings are, if you will, "digested" by the sponsor and returned to the addict in a more tolerable form. Hopefully the patient will learn to tolerate a broader range of feelings without feeling overwhelmed or threatened and without falling back into more primitive defenses like dissociation.

The goal of working through the Twelve Step process is not to relive traumatic experiences; the goal is to begin to tolerate a range of feelings in the presence of another trusted person without reverting to old ways of experiencing emotions. This process of learning to trust others in a reciprocal relationship, without being harmed, helps addicts develop what psychologists call *boundaries.*

Boundaries and Emotional Growth

The Twelve Step model encompasses far more than what meets the eye. The Twelve Steps have long been appreciated for how they help people dramatically improve their lives, but I like to take the relevance of the Twelve Steps one step further. In the following pages, you will see how working the Twelve Step recovery process actually aligns with "repairing" the brain functions that trauma interrupts.

I greatly admire the work of Peter Fonagy and his associates. In the following discussion I'll talk about how Fonagy's thinking on boundaries and trauma relate to addiction. You'll also see how profoundly effective the Twelve Steps are in helping addicts restore trusting relationships and healthy boundaries, despite the ruptures of childhood trauma.[10]

Let's focus for a moment on how the mere availability of another person creates the possibility of emotional growth. We will explore why boundaries are so important to this process. As background, let's look at how infant/parent interactions relate to this process. When infants enter the world, they merely *are;* they are awash in feelings that they are unable to identify or regulate. Eventually, each child evolves into a conscious, self-aware being.

The "self" evolves as the result of complex interactions between the environment and the genetic endowment of the child. Infant research has shown that initially the child is completely interested in activities that are perfectly "contingent," or conditional, upon his or her mind. Those naturally occurring activities, those that are most contingent, are contained within his or her body boundaries. For instance, the child likes watching his or her limbs move.

At around six months of age, the child becomes interested in activities that are close but "imperfectly contingent," or nearly contingent, upon the child's mind. At this age, the child is interested in moving his or her hands to strike a mobile or roll a ball. Because a child's brain has large areas dedicated to the assessment of other human faces, sure enough, the child also likes seeing responses in the faces of other humans, particularly that of a parent or primary caregiver.

The reactions of others are "imperfectly contingent" upon the child, the child's actions, and even the child's feelings. When a child is hurt or angry, the child runs to his or her mother and anticipates a reaction—perhaps of sympathy or comfort. The child is particularly aware of the responses portrayed on the face of the caregiver.

Studies have looked at how primary caregivers respond to children who are having emotional experiences. We are, after all, a "mimetic" species. While you might expect that a caregiver would mimic or mirror the child's feelings, studies have shown that something more subtle happens. Caregivers actually exaggerate with marked facial expressions what they perceive the feeling to be in the child. The caregiver is signaling an appreciation of the child's feelings without actually taking on that state. Although the caregiver does not allow the child's feeling states to invade the caregiver's own, he or she helps the child place a *boundary* around feelings.[11]

The caregiver is providing what we might call "pretend states," or exaggerated facial expressions of the child's emotional experience. There is good evidence that this is the primary means of how we come to know our own emotions. In addition, the caregiver also offers genuine emotional benefits to the child beyond simply mirroring the child's feelings. For example, if a child is hurt or angry, and the mother actually takes on that same emotional state, it would neither help the child identify his or her feelings nor help the child be soothed. It would only make the child feel worse. In a healthy interaction with a caregiver, the child is allowed to identify feelings and tap into the caregiver's more developed range of emotions and maturity for comfort.

This process can go awry in many ways when the child repeatedly triggers negative feelings in the caregiver. A child may start suppressing feelings and focus on managing the caregiver's feelings to avoid future dangerous, frightening feelings. Or a more serious outcome, the child learns that his or her feelings exist in the other, outside his or her body boundaries. Psychiatrists call this "projective identification," when the only way to have a feeling is to experience it in the other. This tendency can be seen in patients with borderline personality disorder and those with post-traumatic stress disorder. This is a state in which boundaries tend to be very poorly maintained.

Boundaries and Addiction

Poor boundaries and being responsible for the feelings of others is a common feature of family members living with active addiction. Dr. Stephanie Brown will explain these family dynamics in chapter 5. When a child lives with an alcoholic parent, the child may not get his or her emotional needs met. Instead, that child may need to focus on negotiating a family system where survival requires the child to avoid triggering negative feelings in a parent. That child may even need to try to monitor or contain a parent's use of drugs or alcohol. This is a typical scenario for codependency to develop.

Another emotional trap happens when a parent either cannot understand or misreads a child's emotional experiences.

The parent may try to appreciate the child's experience but still superimposes his or her own interpretation. When the parent is unable to identify and reflect back the child's feelings, perhaps because of the parent's own developmental issues, the child may never develop a robust connection between his or her primary feelings and the second-order representation of those feelings based on the reflected appreciation of his or her feelings by others. This child may grow into an adult who later complains of feeling empty and has great difficulty experiencing feelings as genuine.

Neglect is perhaps the most serious of all problems that derail emotional development. A neglected child is not even offered the opportunity to get what he or she needs to mature, leaving large areas of the brain underdeveloped and poorly integrated, particularly the anterior cingulate and orbiofrontal regions. As I mentioned earlier, even a relatively healthy path of emotional growth can be ruptured and aborted by trauma. Trauma can leave a child unable to develop mutual relationships with others. The child is then left to rely on underdeveloped, more primitive means of dealing with his or her feelings.

One of the greatest benefits of the Twelve Step process is how addicts learn to re-establish the process of healthy relationships. This is where a sponsor becomes especially important. Sponsees learn, in the course of this relationship, that they can have feelings without triggering overwhelming reactions in the sponsor. They learn to trust that a sponsor will not abandon or abuse them. The recovering individual also learns that he or she can have strong feelings without invading or harming the sponsor. This sponsor relationship is a crash course in helping an addict form a boundary around his or her experiences.

As recovery progresses, the now-sober addict becomes a sponsor to other addicts, further developing a mature sense of boundaries. A sponsor will begin to practice the experience of providing others with facial expressions signaling his or her appreciation of their feelings without being invaded by those feelings. Sponsors do not need to rescue their sponsees from pain or shame. By rescuing, sponsors will learn that they just make the sponsee dependent on the sponsor to continually manage the feelings. Sponsoring others teaches recovering people the power of simply being available as a source of support, connection, and reflected appreciation.

Sponsors learn to maintain a sense of caring detachment from others: being available without being overwhelmed by others' problems.

Guidelines for Taking
Prescription Pain Medication

Chances are you picked up this book because you are concerned about how you or someone close to you is using pain medication. In discussing guidelines for proper use of medication, it's important to first determine if an abuse or addiction problem exists. The following signs indicate problem use of pain medication:

- You are using someone else's prescription.
- You are obtaining drugs from an illicit source or by illegal means.
- You are no longer using the drug for the symptoms for which it was originally prescribed.
- You need the drug in order to function.
- You are obtaining the medication from multiple physicians.
- You withhold information, such as a history of alcoholism or addiction, from your physician.

- You are lying about or hiding your use.
- You are cited for driving under the influence.
- Your friends, family members, or co-workers have expressed concern.
- You are advised to stop but don't or won't.
- You are preoccupied about your medication, focused on the next dose, and concerned about procurement (how you will get more).
- You fill your prescriptions sooner than would be expected and make excuses for why.
- Your medication is causing you to withdraw from previously enjoyable and productive activities, even though your pain has been adequately controlled.
- You are making excuses for, rationalizing, or denying your use.

Assessing Your Risk for Addiction to Pain Medication

The following questions can help you to assess your risk for addiction to pain medication.

- Have you ever been addicted to drugs or alcohol? If you have, you should realize that you will readily become addicted to opiates regardless of what your drug of addiction has been.
- Do you have a first-degree relative—parent, sibling, or child—with addiction or alcoholism? If you do, your risk for having this genetic potential is roughly 50 percent.
- Have you ever thought that you could become addicted to something or have you ever described yourself as having an "addictive personality"?
- Are you a trauma survivor?

If the answer to any of these questions is "yes" and you have a well-defined need for pain medication, you should be in the care of a physician with expertise in addiction medicine.

If you believe you are in trouble with pain medication, the following points are very important:

- Speak to the prescribing doctor immediately and make plans to stop the medication. *Do not stop on your own.*

- If you develop withdrawal symptoms when you stop (such as crushing pain in your low back and legs or feelings of sadness, anxiety, agitation, sleeplessness, or desperation), you may need to be detoxified, possibly in a treatment center.

- If you are already in recovery, speak to your sponsor and increase your meeting attendance. If Twelve Step recovery is not currently a part of your life, be sure your doctor consults with a physician who has experience treating addiction.

If you have an acute need for pain medication, such as after a surgery or severe injury, a good rule of thumb is to never take pain medication for longer than fourteen days.

The risk for triggering addiction and misuse is obviously much greater if you have a previous history of addiction, particularly if that addiction was to opiates. The greatest risk for reactivating addiction is during the first six to twelve months of sobriety. Every effort should be made to avoid any exposure to opiates during this time as it will reawaken all of the distortions, feelings of desperation, and cravings of addiction.

Pain Management for Recovering People

If you are a person in recovery, I recommend the following approach when managing acute pain.

First, tell your surgeon well before the procedure about your history of addiction and develop a plan. Usually I recommend patient-controlled analgesia (PCA), which is an IV unit that allows you to control the amount and frequency of the pain medication. The surgeon needs to realize that you will probably need more medication than the average person, as you will be tolerant to the effects even if you have been sober many years.

Agree with your physician that the duration of the PCA will be for whatever is customary for the procedure, presuming there are no surgical complications. Stop the PCA after that interval. At that point, you will be switched to oral medication.

I recommend at this point that you ask for help from your recovering peers. Have someone from your Twelve Step program help you determine whether you really need pain relief, are anxious, or are anticipating pain. Or is it merely your disease demanding more medication? When you leave the hospital, do not leave with a big bottle of pain medication. Ask for assistance. Make it another person's responsibility to give you daily medication allotments. Make every effort to keep the duration of treatment under fourteen days.

Don't be afraid to consult with a physician who specializes in addiction medicine if you feel you are getting into trouble. Most people get through situations like this without any problem, particularly if they have been sober more than twelve months. I have alcoholic patients who can be very cavalier about these situations. They insist, "I'm not a pill popper" or, "Pills never did anything for me. They are not my thing." In spite of their protests, I have seen many alcoholics become inadvertently addicted to prescription pain medication.

What about chronic pain, what is coming to be called *maladaptive pain?* We are emphasizing in this book an abstinence-based approach to the treatment of pain medication abuse. The key recommendation in this situation is to be sure that you are being cared for by a team of professionals with expertise in the management of pain.

If you have been previously addicted to opiates and you now have uncontrollable maladaptive pain symptoms, I strongly encourage the involvement of an addiction medicine team. This is the best way to protect your abstinence-based recovery.

Conclusion

Recovery is an intense, time-consuming process. It involves a "rewiring" of brain mechanisms. Establishing growth in a firm recovery can take months or even years.

The misuse of prescription pain medication is a terrifically complicated issue. It includes experimentation and abuse by youth, which can be life-threatening if abused with other central nervous system depressants such as alcohol. It can lead to addiction in the genetically predisposed. And opiates are particularly gratifying to individuals who have a history of interpersonal trauma. Pain is a confounding factor.

Patients and physicians can fall into the trap of addiction accidentally in the course of innocent attempts to manage pain. Once the disease is triggered, patients can feel neglected or pushed away by caregivers who should be identifying the problem and developing a plan for treatment. Chronic pain is a confounding condition, and its treatment splinters across several diverse medical approaches. I am an advocate of what I call "pain recovery." When the addictive disease has been identified in a pain patient, the patient needs to be detoxed from opiates and placed in a comprehensive treatment program. In treatment, patients can be encouraged to participate in a Twelve Step experience, which creates the potential for significant emotional growth.

Those of us who work in addiction medicine have all seen remarkable recoveries in patients with chronic pain taking opiates. Pain and addiction are both conditions from which patients can recover. As you read on, you will learn more about the disease of addiction, its influence on families, treatment, and intervention. Prescription pain medication addiction has become a common problem. It requires assistance from diligent and skillful professionals. But rest assured, treatment works.

Now let us turn our attention to addiction treatment. You may have identified a problem with prescription pain medication and you want help. In the next chapter, Dr. Marvin D. Seppala presents a thorough discussion of the basic principles of treatment. If it is a family member you are trying to help, Dr. Robert J. Meyers and Dr. John Gardin provide a discussion of the principles of intervention in chapter 3. William White discusses the history of drug abuse and addiction over the centuries in chapter 4. Dr. Stephanie Brown, in chapter 5, emphasizes the family issues in addiction. Make no mistake, addiction is a family disease and successful treatment requires full participation in the treatment process by the important people in the identified patient's life.

How Addiction Treatment Works

Marvin D. Seppala, M.D.

Carol has just finished her first surgical case of the day and has five to go. She tears off her gloves and gown and retreats to the bathroom, where she swallows ten tablets of Vicodin. She has been using up to sixty tablets of this addictive opioid medication a day for the past three years. Ten tablets will keep her steady and free of withdrawal pain for the rest of the morning. Carol is a successful surgeon, and she is an addict. For the remainder of the day, she will continue her surgical caseload while high on opioids.

Carol has tried to stop using Vicodin on her own. Using her knowledge of opioid detoxification, she has tried to slowly taper the dose, but her best efforts have failed. Tolerance has developed, and she continues to use opioids every few hours to prevent the excruciating pain of withdrawal. The shame related to her behavior and the fear of losing her license prevent her from seeking help. She fears for her job, knowing she is no longer the surgeon she once was. She is bordering on hopelessness; she knows she must quit but cannot do so. At times she contemplates suicide, which appears to be a better option than revealing her secret. She knows the risks she is taking by performing surgery under the influence, but she can't stop.

Why can't Carol just stop? Because she no longer has a choice. Addiction is a disease of the brain characterized by the compulsive, ongoing use of substances in spite of significant adverse consequences. These substances alter brain function, resulting in loss of choice—she must continue to use the drug. The addicted individual can no longer make the decision that seems obvious to the rest of us. The non-addicted person reasons, "Simply stop using the drug and end the negative consequences." But Carol can't make that choice. The drug has, essentially, taken control of her brain. She has lost control of her ability to make decisions about whether or not she uses opioids. Scientific research has shown us that, in fact, brain cells adapt to addictive substances. The cells function differently, disrupting normal brain function, due to regular exposure to drugs of abuse.

The Hijacked Brain

Scientists have now identified receptors in the brain for every major class of addictive substance. Receptors are distinctly matched by size, shape, and function to certain natural chemical messengers called neurotransmitters. The drugs that cause intoxication are chemically related to the neurotransmitters, so the drugs of abuse bind to these receptors in a similar manner—but remarkably they are more powerful in how they affect the brain.

The genetic codes of these receptors have been identified and the receptors have been cloned for study, providing remarkable evidence about how these drugs affect our brain cells. These brain receptors have been located and mapped, identifying the primary region responsible for addiction as the mesolimbic dopamine system.[1]

The mesolimbic dopamine system is the reward center of the brain, which promotes the repetition of pleasurable activities. This area is subcortical (beneath the cortex), therefore beneath the level of conscious thought. Thus, the primary part of the brain involved in our response to intoxicants is not under the control of our conscious thought, and once addiction occurs, this area takes over to drive the individual to continue to seek the drug.

Carol's use of opioids is out of her control. Carol, like other addicts, has undergone a re-prioritization of her drives. Drives are the innate motivations that define our most basic behaviors. The most powerful drive is for survival itself. Human drives also include nutritional intake, fluid intake, and social interaction. Humans rarely undermine these basic instincts for survival, but addiction pushes humans into catastrophic behaviors.

If you've lived with an alcoholic or addict, you probably have seen how family and career obligations always take the backseat to addiction. People in the grips of addiction, in fact, seem to have no concerns about their own safety or health. For example, consider the heroin addict who uses a dirty needle with someone else's blood left in it. This addict is risking life itself to get high.

Or consider Jeff, a twenty-eight-year-old alcoholic with pancreatitis. He left the hospital hours after having surgery to treat pancreatic cysts. Tubes were sticking out of the surgical wound and hooked up to a vacuum pump to drain the cysts so they would heal correctly. He unhooked the apparatus himself and left the hospital in his gown, with the tubes dangling from his abdomen, to go to the nearest bar to find a drink. He admitted that he had no idea if this was a dangerous act or not. He was not able to rationally think through his situation because addiction had taken over his brain, and craving drove him to seek alcohol. His primary drive after major surgery was not survival—it was the addiction.

Addiction As a Disease

Addiction is defined as a disease by the American Medical Association, the American Psychiatric Association, and the World Health Organization. One definition of disease suggests the following criteria. The condition of addiction

- has a clear biologic basis
- is marked by identifiable signs and symptoms
- shows a predictable course and outcome
- is not caused by volitional acts or by choice[2]

It has been established that addiction is a disease of the brain and researchers have identified the specific areas of the brain involved, thus a biologic basis for addiction exists. The *Diagnostic and Statistical Manual of Mental Disorders (DSM)* of the American Psychiatric Association describes the symptoms of all psychiatric illness, including those of addiction, which is referred to as psychoactive substance dependence.

The signs and symptoms of addiction include

- withdrawal symptoms
- tolerance
- using more of a substance than intended
- unsuccessful attempts to control use
- much time spent in obtaining, using, or recovering from the effects of use
- use despite adverse consequences

I mentioned earlier how the brain is altered, below the level of consciousness, to allow the addictive behaviors to manifest. Thus, we have a disease that begins with a conscious decision to use intoxicants. However, once the brain is hijacked, a person is driven to continue to use substances by powerful subconscious factors associated with abnormal stimulation of the pleasure center of the brain. The individual no longer has control over the behavior. Addiction is not the result of volitional acts or choice. Therefore, addiction meets all the criteria for disease.

Learned Behavior or Moral Issue?

Some people argue that addiction isn't a disease; they believe that addiction is a learned behavior that can be addressed by learning other adaptive behaviors. Carol certainly made conscious decisions to start using opioids, and she learned that they made her feel better and relieved pain. But she also made a decision to stop using Vicodin. She has tried to stop, but she cannot. Jeff would have been better off sitting in his hospital bed after surgery, but he risked his life to drink. Both Carol and Jeff are no longer able to control their use of these substances because the disease of addiction manifests in the brain regions that are below the level of conscious thought.

Addiction is also considered by some to be a moral issue, and addicts are described as self-indulgent. One can examine animal studies for further consideration of the nature of addiction as disease. Rats can be ordered from laboratory supply companies that represent different strains of addiction. There are rats available that do not drink, rats that drink but can take it or leave it, and rats that will drink until they die. If allowed to breed within the strain, all the progeny of these rats will drink or not, just like their parents.

Since rats have not been described as having morals, or to be self-indulgent, one has to consider the possibility that these animals have a biologically determined behavior. As mentioned, there are research rats that, if allowed to, will drink themselves to death. Like humans, rats are so susceptible to the power of addiction that their survival instincts will be undermined by this disease.

Out of Choices

Carol is eventually asked to meet with her department chairperson. When she arrives at the meeting, she discovers that representatives of the state board of medical examiners are also present. She is told that members of the department have been quite concerned about her during the past year. The people she is meeting with describe reports of substandard performance, inadequate record keeping, and erratic mood swings, and they say she was not available for phone calls from nurses on a regular basis, even when she was on call.

The department chairperson has known Carol for ten years and voices his concern about her performance, as well as about the divorce she endured two years ago, the loss of her two children who are with her ex-husband, her isolation from old friends, and her lack of involvement in the department.

The chairperson has also been tracking the narcotic samples in her office during the past couple months, which has revealed undocumented losses of Vicodin. Office staff told the investigators that they were aware that Carol was ordering the Vicodin, but they had no idea what had become of it. Carol is desperate to protect her reputation and her livelihood, so she tells them the maintenance staff must have stolen it. She says she saw a janitor leaving the office in a suspicious manner.

The group is not persuaded by her argument, and they ask her to provide a urine sample for a drug screen. Carol used Vicodin that day and she knows it will show up. She tries to postpone the test and then lashes out in anger. How dare they accuse her of stealing drugs? But they don't back down, and they tell her she needs help. Carol breaks down and admits to taking a Vicodin now and then, minimizing the extent of the problem. She provides the urine sample and agrees to an addiction evaluation.

Types of Treatment

Three primary types of treatment are available in the United States. Depending on one's insurance coverage, the decision facing most people in need of addiction treatment will be whether to enter a residential facility or to attend an outpatient treatment program. Opioid addicts have a third treatment option, the use of maintenance therapy, which is the use of medication to eliminate the craving for the opioid.

Residential Treatment

The current model of residential treatment began at Hazelden, located in Center City, Minnesota. Hazelden opened in the late 1940s and developed what eventually came to be called the Minnesota Model, which continues to be the primary treatment model used throughout the world. The Minnesota Model is based on the Twelve Steps of Alcoholics Anonymous and uses a multidisciplinary team to provide addiction treatment services. Abstinence from all addicting substances is emphasized, and individuals are held accountable for their past behavior and their recovery.

Both residential and outpatient treatments are effective in addressing addiction and alcoholism. Residential treatment, however, offers certain advantages, which include

- providing an immersion experience into recovery
- insulating the individual from the addictive substances

- immediately limiting further damage to the family
- providing more time for therapy and peer interaction

Residential treatment provides more of the necessary services for the multiple problems facing a recovering addict. Residential treatment also appears to be better suited for people who have extreme addictions, certain medical and psychiatric problems, and little social support for abstinence. These groups have better outcomes in residential treatment, but people with less severe problems do just as well in outpatient care.

Professionals, such as pilots and physicians, who can place the public at risk with ongoing use of drugs and alcohol may be better off in residential treatment. However, residential treatment is expensive and disruptive to the workplace and the family.

Outpatient Treatment

Medical and economic factors resulted in an expansion of outpatient treatment in the late 1980s and early 1990s. In 2002, 85 percent of those entering addiction treatment attended outpatient programs, as these programs are more available, less expensive, and less disruptive to the workplace and the family.[3]

Outpatient treatment services are usually offered two to three hours a day, several times per week. The programs are set up with day and evening hours, making them easily accessible. The services are more intense and frequent initially, perhaps for the first month, then diminish over time. Treatment lasts for six to twelve weeks, but it can last for up to a year or more. The treatment itself is based on the same principles as residential treatment, and it is as effective as residential treatment for those with less severe illness. Outpatient treatment, however, lacks the extensive variety of services and multi-disciplinary team members available in residential care.

Outpatient programs have a higher drop-out rate, and they lend themselves to more drug and alcohol use during the treatment experience. Participants attend treatment while remaining in the environment in which they were using drugs and alcohol, which can be very difficult without proper support. These and other factors need to be weighed when choosing a treatment program.

Maintenance Therapy

Maintenance therapy is limited to treatment of opioid addiction, primarily addiction to heroin, but it can be used to treat addiction to OxyContin and other prescription pain medications. Maintenance therapy uses a medication within the same class as the addicting drug to prevent intoxication, withdrawal, and illicit use. This is very effective at eliminating the use of heroin and opioids and decreasing illegal activities and medical problems such as hepatitis C and HIV infection.

The most common medication used for maintenance therapy of opioid addiction is methadone, which can only be obtained at methadone clinics. Buprenorphine was released as a maintenance therapy in 2002 and has the distinct advantage of being prescribed in the privacy of a physician's office. Although these two medications are opioids and can be abused, specific restrictions are in place to limit this as much as possible.

Medications are also used to complement traditional treatment programs. Only a few medications have been shown to be beneficial, and this is an area of tremendous medical research. These medications help reduce cravings for the addictive drug, thus promoting abstinence. The research on anti-craving and anti-addiction drugs is not complete, and we have much to learn, such as whom these medications are best suited for, but there is great promise. Naltrexone is used to treat both alcohol dependence and opioid dependence. It is effective in limiting the use of alcohol, which can enhance the individual's chances of remaining abstinent. It blocks opiate receptors in the brain and therefore is used for the treatment of opioid dependence.[4] Once someone has started naltrexone and uses an opioid, he or she will not get high from the opioid, thus limiting the person's use.

Antabuse has been used for the treatment of alcohol dependence since the late 1940s. Antabuse causes an adverse reaction when people ingest alcohol, thus preventing use. Antabuse has not been very effective, primarily due to poor adherence to the medication. People just quit taking it before they return to drinking alcohol. This is the problem with all medications: they require monitoring systems to make sure people actually take them.

Acamprosate is a medication available in Europe for the treatment of alcohol dependence. Studies are promising and suggest it may be effective in reducing craving for alcohol, thus reducing relapse.

Medications alone are not the answer for addiction, but they may play a significant role in reducing relapse when combined with traditional addiction treatment. They can reduce the incidence of relapse while people learn the new skills to avoid risk and enhance their ability to remain abstinent. Most relapses occur within the first year after a treatment experience, so anything that can help eliminate relapse during this period can be of great benefit to recovery.[5]

Ending the Addictive Cycle

The primary goal of addiction treatment is to put an end to the cycle of addictive behaviors. This means more than abstinence from the offending substances. When addiction becomes the focus of the person's life, it overshadows all other aspects of life: physical, mental, vocational, family, and social. For this reason, addiction is referred to as a bio-psycho-social disease and a multidisciplinary approach is used to address it. These problems often occur without recognition on the part of the addicted individual. The compulsion is so powerful that he or she can neither see the consequences nor witness the extent of the deterioration. The individual knows there is a problem, can sometimes even admit it is addiction, but fails to see the whole picture.

The problems extend well beyond the use of the drug. Addicts consistently numb themselves with drugs, which limits their ability to witness the whole tragedy. This is more than denial. It is compulsive drug seeking, beneath the level of conscious thought, driving them to continue to use despite the consequences. This is why treatment programs must assess and provide care for addictive behaviors and associated problems to ensure abstinence.

Intermittently, Carol has experienced a degree of recognition that she has a problem, and she now has a new motivation: to maintain her job and her license to practice medicine. The evaluation is difficult because she is so ashamed of using Vicodin throughout the workday and during surgery, and she does not want to admit that her drug use contributed to the divorce and loss of custody of her children. She does not tell her counselor the whole story; it is just too hard to admit.

Carol's evaluation team contacts her department chairperson, some of her peers, the nurses she works with, her friends, and even her ex-husband to gather information. When Carol hears the story from others, she breaks down crying in her counselor's office. But she also begins to see the truth of the addiction.

Carol lost her marriage and her children after her ex-husband refused to lie about her absences from work and social events. She admits to performing surgery while under the influence of opioids and even making mistakes as a result. She has been isolated from friends and family. It is very difficult to admit these things, due to her overwhelming shame, but she finally tells her counselor some of the things she has actually done. The evaluation results in a diagnosis of opioid dependence and a recommendation for treatment. She wants help and agrees to stay in the treatment program.

By the end of the discussion with her counselor, Carol had been without Vicodin for six hours and is beginning to show signs of withdrawal. The counselor notes this and sends her directly for a physical examination. She is immediately given medication to alleviate the opioid withdrawal symptoms. The exam reveals no significant medical problems, but her laboratory tests show liver damage from the acetaminophen in Vicodin and the urine drug screen shows opioids. She will have more tests to follow up on the liver damage later in her treatment.

Carol has described occasional thoughts of suicide and is seen by a psychologist and a psychiatrist. She is very sad but has no ongoing thoughts of suicide, so they agree to monitor the depressive symptoms to see whether they are caused by her addiction or by a depressive illness. Carol is exhausted but relieved. She has finally admitted her problem to someone else and can get the help she needs.

A Thorough Evaluation

The care of someone with addictive disease begins in the same manner as the care of any disease—with evaluation of the problem and establishment of a diagnosis. A thorough initial evaluation is necessary to determine that addiction exists, the extent of the addiction, any other medical or psychiatric problems, and whether medical detoxification is necessary. Information is gathered from the client and from any prior and current medical and psychiatric caregivers.

Some people are hesitant to provide the entire history of their drug use and others cannot recall the details, so evaluations can include contact with the addict's family members, friends, co-workers, probation officer, attorney, and employer. The evaluation team, counselor, or physician will use the information to make a diagnosis specific to the type of drug used. A physical examination and laboratory testing are needed to determine if any other medical problems are present.

Most treatment programs use a series of psychological tests and a psychological evaluation to examine if any mental health problems need to be addressed. Psychiatrists are available for evaluation and care of significant psychiatric illness. All of the evaluations are pulled together to form a treatment plan that defines the initial addiction treatment. This plan is updated as the client's condition changes.

Addiction treatment addresses multiple issues to foster abstinence and to establish the foundation for a healthy, productive life. Treatment is very complicated as a result of the numerous problems that require evaluation and attention.

Remember, addiction affects all aspects of a person's life: physical, mental, vocational, family, and social. Good treatment provides the necessary care at the right time. Some of the problems need immediate attention, like detoxification. Other problems, such as an addictive lifestyle, must be addressed during treatment. Still other issues require attention both throughout the treatment experience and afterward, such as the healing of a family.

Detoxification

Carol's opioid detoxification is uncomplicated. She feels minor discomfort, but it is remarkably better than her own attempts to detoxify at home. She spends her first week of treatment on a medical unit so she can be closely monitored. She is anxious and can't sleep for several nights, but this improves and she starts to feel healthier. It takes ten days to get through the detoxification, and by then she is actively involved in treatment.

Detoxification is a medical procedure used to prevent withdrawal symptoms and provide a safe and comfortable transition to a drug-free state. Detoxification differs by the class of drug that has been used and is often complicated due to the regular use of more than one class of drug. For example, someone who uses alcohol and an opioid on a daily basis would need separate, but simultaneous, detoxification from both. Some people confuse detoxification with treatment itself, but detox is only the beginning.

Eliminating the drug from an addict's system is necessary, but extreme vulnerability to relapse follows because craving is incredibly strong at the point of discontinuation. After detoxification, the drug is no longer the problem, but the long-term changes to the brain of the addict and psychosocial problems must be addressed. Therefore, the treatment of addiction does not require separation into drug-specific groups; cocaine addicts, alcoholics, and prescribed-opioid addicts can be addressed in a similar, but not identical, manner.

Cracking through Denial

Using the individual's internal strength and motivation is important to the start of the treatment experience. Rather than confronting the negative aspects of an addict's situation, a good counselor trained in what is called "motivational enhancement" techniques will support him or her in pursuing help for the problems he or she has begun to recognize. This eliminates conflict and enhances motivation for treatment. The decision to care for oneself is ultimately up to the individual.

Motivational enhancement establishes a therapeutic relationship with the counselor rather than a confrontational relationship. Addicts need help with a number of problems, and the goal of treatment personnel is to provide the necessary assistance. People in the midst of addiction rarely recognize all of their problems or the degree of their dysfunction, due to the nature of this brain disease.

They do know something is wrong, however, and a good counselor can prompt further recognition. When addicts begin to truly recognize how deeply addiction has affected their lives, a good counselor can also help motivate addicts toward putting their lives back together. Recognition of addictive behaviors and associated problems enhances understanding, which influences motivation and provides a positive initiation to the treatment experience.

Eliminating Addictive Behaviors

The primary goal of addiction treatment is to eliminate addictive behaviors. Addiction treatment consists of therapy, education, and fellowship. These experiences are intended to address addictive behaviors, help the individual recognize the problems in his or her life, and provide the skills to address these problems and maintain abstinence. This is accomplished by activities that establish and support abstinence from drugs and alcohol. Initially, this requires a strict focus on the addiction itself, as the individual's brain is still under the residual influence of addicting substances and those substances have become the single most important factor in his or her life. Addicts in early treatment recognize the degree to which they are out of control.

Group Therapy

In group therapy, people are able to see in other addicts the very issues they cannot admit to themselves. This breaks down defenses and opens people's minds to the possibility that they are actually experiencing the same problems they see in others. The intended focus of group therapy is on abstinence, but because addicts experience deterioration in so many aspects of life, the groups could deal with a wide variety of topics. Such topics include

- the physical consequences of addiction
- how drug and alcohol use affected the family
- honesty
- how to use the support of others to address new problems
- how to deal with the losses caused by addictive behavior

Honest sharing and intimacy are emphasized in such groups. These people not only recognize their own problems in the stories of others but also discover a profound sense of acceptance by others, in spite of their behaviors. In group therapy, addicts begin to recognize they are not unique or alone; others understand what they've been through and can be of help. Group therapy also breaks isolation so often associated with addiction. As people interact in a group setting, they begin to develop new relationships, share intimacies, and establish friendships, all of which can improve social functioning.

Group therapy also prepares people for Twelve Step meetings so they will at least be somewhat comfortable in a group setting.

Individual Therapy

Individual therapy is also used in addiction treatment. Each client is assigned a counselor who provides guidance and insight into addictive behaviors and the activities associated with healing in early recovery. These counselors are often, but not always, in recovery from addiction themselves. They provide the knowledge of recovery and the Twelve Steps needed by their clients to remain abstinent and to begin to change their behaviors. Counselors actually act as role models for the changes their clients will need to make to start living drug free.

Individual therapy may also be needed to address private issues and certain mental health problems. If a patient is having flashbacks of sexual assault or is extremely depressed, an individual therapist with specific expertise in trauma or mental health issues is critical in helping this patient. This level of psychotherapy requires a psychologist, psychiatrist, or social worker. Although it could be appropriate for the individual to address such a topic in a group, these issues are usually assigned to individual therapy. Individual therapy is also necessary for those who cannot easily open up in a group setting. Such decisions depend on the treatment setting and the individual's situation.

Education

In treatment, patients are educated about addiction as a brain disease, what to expect in early abstinence, and how to re-enter the "real world." Education is usually in the form of lectures and reading assignments, which are provided to give people in treatment a clear understanding of the problems they are facing. The more informed people are, the better they can advocate for themselves and the more they understand what is necessary to maintain abstinence.

Carol has a good medical education but little understanding of addiction. She sees addiction as a personal failing, a moral problem, and she sees herself as a horribly flawed person. She is so ashamed of her behavior that she cannot admit to anyone that she performed surgery under the influence.

Before treatment, Carol had no idea that her brain had been hijacked by the opioids and that she could not count on rational thinking to address her use. It has helped a great deal to begin to understand how she changed due to the addiction. She now knows it wasn't her intent to act in the way she did—she did not want to be an addict or ruin her family and her job—but she seemed to do it without choice. The education about addiction has provided her with an explanation for her behavior and some hope needed for her future without drugs.

Fellowship

Fellowship plays an integral role in the treatment process as well. People in the midst of addiction treatment and in early recovery need help from each other—they may be the best teachers and role models for both what works and what does not. The fellowship experienced in a treatment setting provides a level of intimacy that may have become foreign to the addict. They need to re-establish intimacy and positive relationships. They need the acceptance, understanding, and experience of another addict as a sounding board for their shame, guilt, and fears.

Often people will describe past experiences or share their innermost fears of recovery to a trusted peer, even though they are unwilling to share this information with anyone else. Twelve Step recovery is founded on the stories of addiction and healing told to one another. These stories provide needed information about how other people have stayed clean and sober, and they elicit hope, a necessary component to early recovery.

Treatment programs offer unstructured time to promote fellowship that can establish the bond of friendship found when sharing such a common experience. Carol entered treatment believing she was the only female physician addicted to opioids in the western hemisphere. In treatment, she met other physicians and other women with addiction and alcoholism, even a female internist who was using Vicodin and OxyContin. When Carol discovered how similar her experience was to theirs, she was flooded with relief and a surprising sense of hope.

Breaking the Isolation

Carol finds group therapy to be very difficult at first. She has been isolated and has not yet revealed any of her problems to other people. She is a surgeon and has witnessed extreme illness, trauma, and death without having to talk to people about it. She doesn't believe this kind of treatment will be of help to her. She wonders how talking about her problems can relieve her of this compulsion.

Carol cannot imagine sharing her personal failings in a public arena. She doesn't trust some of the group members, and she doesn't like the counselor who provokes her peers to expose their failings and their feelings about themselves. Carol even dismisses the counselor because she isn't a medical doctor. In spite of this bias, she finds the stories of her peers to be extremely familiar and, at times, gut wrenching. She starts to experience the pain of her own experiences as she listens to others talk about theirs.

One day in group, Carol begins to cry as another addicted mother speaks of her divorce and the loss of custody of her children due to active addiction. It is the turning point for Carol as she admits to the painful feelings and shame associated with her divorce, especially now that her children live with their father. This admission and the expression of her pain allow her to begin to describe to her peers the other areas of her life that are haunting her. She admits to the use of Vicodin during surgery and the tremendous fear of causing harm to patients who had come to her for help.

Carol is beginning the process of recovery by admitting her problems, examining them, and talking them out. She is feeling the pain associated with her addiction rather than avoiding and numbing it. She starts to feel less depressed, and after a psychiatric evaluation, she learns that her depression, even the thoughts of suicide, were induced by the opioids and her remorse, not by a separate depressive illness.

Carol even begins to laugh on occasion, something she has not done naturally in years. She finds that the other women are of great help to her, and she truly enjoys their company and their support. She begins to believe that she can get clean and sober and establish a good life based on the Twelve Steps.

Twelve Step Recovery

The Twelve Steps of Alcoholics Anonymous (AA) and Narcotics Anonymous (NA) are used in most treatment programs in the United States. Research has documented that people involved in AA after treatment are more likely to remain abstinent than those who are not involved in AA.[6] The founders of AA realized that addicts had a physical reaction to alcohol different from non-addicts, and that they needed a spiritual approach to life in order to address the wreckage of their past, improve their lives, and stay sober. The Twelve Steps are reprinted on page 169 of this book.

The first five Steps are those primarily used in addiction treatment programs. Step One is "We admitted we were powerless over alcohol—that our lives had become unmanageable." Without this Step, without acceptance of this disease, the individual has no foundation from which to start to heal and change. This may sound simple, but it is remarkably difficult for people to admit that they have a problem and that they can no longer control or predict their use of addicting substances. Ultimately, getting an addict or alcoholic to recognize his or her problem is a primary objective of addiction treatment programs.

Step Two states "Came to believe that a Power greater than ourselves could restore us to sanity." It reveals the spiritual solution associated with the Twelve Steps. It is not a dogmatic approach, but insists that individuals determine a power greater than themselves, which will be of help to them. This might be "God" or even the Twelve Step group they attend. The emphasis is on getting outside of oneself for the answers to this problem.

The Third Step states "Made a decision to turn our will and our lives over to the care of God *as we understood Him.*" Step Three is an expansion of the concept of a spiritual solution. It asks a person to begin a process of self-examination based on spiritual principles.

Steps Four and Five state "Made a searching and fearless moral inventory of ourselves" and "Admitted to God, to ourselves, and to another human being the exact nature of our wrongs." These Steps provide the opportunity for self-evaluation. A person does an inventory, which begins the process of addressing the shame and guilt associated with past behaviors. This is a difficult undertaking, but the results, when done correctly, are remarkable. Steps Four and Five provide the first sense of healing from the damage caused by addictive behaviors and help to relieve excessive guilt and shame.

The Twelve Steps provide a framework for recovery that can be used for a lifetime. Initiation to the Twelve Steps during treatment makes for an easy transition to Twelve Step program attendance after treatment.

Overcoming Resistance

Carol is perplexed by the use of the Twelve Steps to treat a disease. She is agnostic and resists the use of a spirituality to address her addiction. She has found the First Step to be very helpful in fully examining the consequences of her use and admitting to addiction. But then she stalls. She can't get past the spiritual approach presented by the staff.

Fortunately, Carol meets other women who have experienced the same problem. They tell her to think of the peers she trusts as a power greater than herself, to use the group consciousness as a voice of reason. She tries this and finds that she can easily do so with the women she has come to know so well, women with whom she has shared her innermost secrets. Carol uses the women as a sounding board for recovery-related decisions and finds that they care for her and have her best interests in mind. This becomes clear when she is thinking of talking with the medical board about returning to work before her counselor recommends it.

Carol wants to return to work as soon as possible, but her peers tell her she does not seem ready to be exposed to the stress and the potential for relapse. They also tell her she should trust her counselor who has provided constructive guidance up to this point in her treatment. Carol relents, which provides more time for stabilization in recovery. Later, Carol thanks her peers for helping her make the correct decision. She begins to see the merit in using a power greater than herself.

Relapse Preventive Measures

Carol is addicted to opioids, but because she was referred to an abstinence-based treatment program, maintenance therapy (discussed on pages 39–40) was not considered an option. However, her state medical board requires all physicians in recovery from opioids to use naltrexone for several years while being monitored by a diversion program. The board has had positive outcomes with this medication as a deterrent to relapse. That means Carol has no choice if she wants to continue to practice medicine. She decides that using naltrexone is a reasonable requirement, especially if it helps her avoid relapse and save her career.

Gender Issues

Carol is in a gender-specific treatment program. There are men and women in the program at the same time, but because they live in separate units or wards, they rarely interact with one another. This separation is of benefit to both sexes, although it is not used by all treatment programs. Gender-specific programs are more commonly found in residential facilities, but some outpatient programs are based on gender. The real advantages are found in group therapy. Single gender groups can more easily address gender and sexual issues. Mixed gender groups tend to have a constant battle with sexual tension.

Group therapy in treatment involves vulnerable individuals who have just given up addictive substances and destructive behaviors, including sexual issues. The sexual issues run the gamut from sexual abuse to sexual promiscuity and sexual compulsivity. As people share their past problems and their feelings, they become closer and share a level of intimacy. Inevitably, in mixed gender groups, sexual romances develop because they distract people from focusing on addiction treatment. Rather than concentrating on their addiction and the difficulties of treatment, the group members become absorbed in one another. Obviously, it feels tremendously better to be in love than it does to spill your guts about how addiction has destroyed your family.

Women also experience addiction differently than men. There is a higher degree of stigma associated with female alcoholics and drug addicts. The course of the disease of alcoholism develops more rapidly in women than men. This is described as "telescoping," a phenomenon in which the time taken by women to go from the initiation of heavy drinking to major problems is shorter than that of men.

Women are also more susceptible to alcohol-related medical disorders than men. They develop alcohol-related cirrhosis,[7] cardiomyopathy,[8] and brain impairment[9] at the same rate as men, despite lower levels of alcohol consumption. Women in addiction treatment have at least twice the rate of mental disorders than those in the general population. They are also more likely than addicted men to have co-existing mental disorders. Compared to men, women need more specialized services—in particular, more mental health services.

On the other hand, women are much more skilled than men at having intimate conversations, expressing feelings, and discussing personal issues with others. As a result, group therapy is a significantly different process for women than for men. In spite of these differences, which support the use of gender-specific treatment, women have the same general treatment outcomes as men.[10]

Mental Health Issues

Co-existing mental disorders complicate the treatment of addiction. This condition is referred to in many ways, such as *co-existing, co-morbid, MI/CD* (mental illness/chemical dependency), and *dual diagnosis*. These terms all mean the same thing and describe someone who has addiction and at least one other major mental disorder.

The rate of co-existing mental disorders among patients in residential treatment facilities is at least 60 percent. These programs should actually be referred to as co-existing or dual diagnosis programs to reflect the primary population receiving treatment. Good residential treatment programs provide mental health services that are integrated into addiction treatment. Outpatient programs may provide some of these services, but in most cases, they will have resources available in the community to which they refer.

Psychological testing and an evaluation by a psychologist are standard in residential treatment facilities. Psychiatrists should be available for evaluation and care throughout the treatment experience. Individual psychotherapy may be offered by psychiatrists, psychologists, and social workers. These mental health professionals should have the ability to incorporate their knowledge of addiction and the treatment of mental disorders to provide the appropriate care for the co-existing illness.

Addiction can mimic a mental disorder, and when they co-exist, the problems related to each are magnified. Stimulants, like cocaine and methamphetamine, can cause psychosis. The mood swings associated with drug use can appear to be bipolar disorder, and drugs can cause symptoms of depression from their use or during withdrawal.

Alcohol can cause depression from chronic use and anxiety from withdrawal. Opioids can cause depressive symptoms during use and anxiety during withdrawal. If someone has depressive illness and is an alcoholic, the alcohol—a depression-inducing substance—will give brief relief from the depression during intoxication, but it will cause worsening symptoms from chronic use.

Depression and Suicide

Most people who enter alcoholism treatment have depressive symptoms, in fact 60 to 80 percent of people admitted to treatment meet criteria for depressive illness. If they remain in treatment and remain abstinent, this percentage of depression drops within three weeks to 10 to 15 percent, about the same rate of depression found in the general population.[11]

Antidepressants are given to many people during their active use of alcohol and other drugs to treat depressive symptoms, which are often caused by the alcohol or drugs being used or the consequences of such use. Abstinence and support found in treatment alleviates this type of depression, and these medications can be discontinued. A true depressive illness requires standard care during addiction treatment, including antidepressant medication and psychotherapy.

Psychiatric medications are necessary in the treatment of co-existing mental disorders, and they should be provided as needed to those in addiction treatment. There are limits to the types of medications that are safe for those in early recovery, and a psychiatrist trained in addiction medicine is often needed to avoid the mistake of providing potentially addicting medicine.

Suicide is highly correlated with alcohol and drug use; in fact, addiction is an extreme risk factor for completed suicide. Suicide must be considered, assessed, and treated by appropriate mental health professionals in all addiction treatment programs. The client's long-term treatment plan should address any co-existing issues and integrate the addiction recovery program with ongoing mental health care.

A Lifelong Disease

Addiction is a chronic illness that requires long-term care, not a single, acute treatment episode of care. Treatment of chronic illness needs to occur over the span of a person's life to ensure continued abstinence and personal growth. This could mean that six weeks of residential treatment is followed by twelve months at a halfway house, then individual therapy for a few years while attending Twelve Step meetings, with plans to do so for life. Or someone could start in intensive outpatient treatment for a month while initiating involvement in Twelve Step meetings three times a week, then shift to outpatient group twice a week for four months, followed by seven months of weekly group involvement, with the opportunity to meet with a counselor whenever needed for a year, with ongoing Twelve Step attendance.

The key is to engage people in lifelong attention to the recovery process in order to minimize the risk of relapse. Once abstinence has been established as the primary goal and people begin to feel some confidence in their ability to remain drug and alcohol free, they are able to start the process of reconstructing their lives. Much of this can occur in a good Twelve Step program.

Twelve Step programs, however, are no substitute for bona fide care from a professional skilled in treating a co-existing mental health issue. There is also a significant drop-out rate in AA, which could be averted by ongoing professional monitoring. The point is, recovering addicts do have specific continuing-care needs long after they leave treatment.

A Long-Term Plan

In Carol's case, it would be irresponsible to simply provide her with detoxification, establish abstinence, and send her directly back into a workplace with ready access to Vicodin. She needs the recovery skills learned in treatment, ongoing support, and a long-term treatment plan to limit her risk of relapse. After residential treatment, Carol's plan is carried out primarily by the state's physician diversion program, which essentially functions as a long-term treatment program. She meets with an addiction counselor once a week, provides a random urine sample once a week to check for drugs of abuse, attends at least three Twelve Step meetings a week, takes naltrexone daily, and sees a therapist to address issues related to the divorce and loss of her children.

Carol is allowed to return to her surgical practice, with restrictions. She can only work forty to fifty hours a week, not eighty to one hundred hours as she had in the past to stay close to her drug supply. She cannot have samples of addictive medications in her office, and she has no access to such medications. She has to have a colleague oversee and co-sign any prescriptions she writes to patients for potentially addicting medications. Carol is also required to have the same physician oversee her involvement in the workplace and report to the diversion program on a monthly basis.

Although Carol readily agreed to all of these requirements when the plan was presented, she really had no choice because she wanted to return to surgery. She learned that her relapse rate was significantly reduced by involvement in the diversion program. While in treatment, she also learned that physicians and pilots involved in such monitoring programs have the highest one-year abstinence rates of any group ever measured—more than 90 percent.[12]

Success rates like these are the result of a long-term treatment program that requires involvement in recovery-related activities. It should also be noted that Carol would not be allowed to practice medicine if she did not agree to these stipulations. The research on these successful programs reveals that professionals from two diverse fields (physicians and pilots) have great recovery rates due to two factors:

- they are highly motivated to keep their jobs
- they are monitored in a manner that requires adherence to a strict treatment regimen over several years

Anyone leaving treatment could benefit from a similar plan, but licensing boards do not exist for most people, so they are left to decide for themselves whether or not to follow the recommendations of the treatment team. Addiction treatment has historically relied on a single treatment episode and expected people to complete it and stay sober for a lifetime. This view is changing dramatically, in large part based on research by Dr. A. Thomas McLellan, who has emphasized the examination and treatment of addiction as a chronic illness.

McLellan has shown that the relapse rates in addiction are very similar to those of other chronic illnesses such as hypertension, asthma, and diabetes.[13] This perspective has helped treatment programs bolster their long-term care systems rather than relying entirely on Twelve Step meetings for all the ongoing needs of their clients. Twelve Step programs are an essential aspect of the long-term plan for the majority of people in recovery, but abstinence over the first twelve to eighteen months of recovery requires additional resources.

Relapse Prevention

Relapse needs to be addressed throughout treatment due to its ongoing serious potential. Addiction has a tremendous hold on people, and the risk of relapse is greatest during the first twelve months after treatment. In fact, only up to 50 percent of people will stay completely abstinent for the first year.[14] Research has shown that the longer the treatment, the better the outcome. This is independent of whether the treatment is provided in a residential setting or on an outpatient basis. Treatment programs that provide a range of services over a twelve- to eighteen-month period will reduce relapse rates compared to shorter programs.

Research has also shown that the people who actually follow their long-term plan are more likely to stay sober than those who do not. The research on AA shows that active involvement—not just attendance—is necessary for better outcomes. People with multiple problems, especially co-existing mental disorders, have lower recovery rates, but treatment of the co-existing disorders improves recovery rates. People who quit smoking or do not smoke have better recovery rates than those who continue to smoke. Addiction professionals use this information to develop relapse prevention plans most likely to result in ongoing abstinence and personal growth.

Returning to the Real World

Carol is home from treatment for a month before the medical board allows her to return to work. During this period, she complies with all of the requirements of her agreement. She enjoys the Twelve Step meetings, makes new friends in recovery, and finds psychotherapy to be helpful. She has enough time to attend to herself and feels fairly confident in her ability to stay clean and sober.

Then Carol returns to work and the daily stress of a surgical practice. She had discussed with her counselor and peers the stress of her job as well as of being back in the "candy store," where she got her drugs, but it did not prepare her for the actual experience. She is frightened that she will be perceived as damaged goods, no longer capable of patient care. She is constantly reminded of Vicodin because she had used it throughout the workplace. She has to work closely with a peer to have prescriptions co-signed, and she feels the shame of her addiction returning.

At first Carol talks to recovering peers at the diversion group and at Twelve Step meetings about her experience, but as she becomes busier and gets back into the routine of work, she begins to keep it to herself. After a month at work, she misses a Twelve Step meeting and does not mention it to her counselor, even though she is required to attend three a week. She is isolating again and begins to feel as if the requirements by the medical board are burdensome and exaggerated. She feels she can stay clean and sober without all the hassles of these meetings. Carol is returning to addictive behaviors— even though she isn't using the drug.

Then one day after a major surgical complication, Carol finds herself in the bathroom with a handful of Vicodin. Before she swallows them, she seems to suddenly awaken and realize what she is about to do. For what seems to be an eternity, Carol is torn between taking the pills and flushing them. She just wants to relieve the pressure, to feel better, and Vicodin has always worked. Suddenly she is reminded of a woman she met at a Twelve Step meeting who told her of a similar struggle after a few months in recovery. Carol recalls how the woman described the hopelessness and desperation of wanting to feel different, but not knowing how. The woman said her struggle ended when she realized she would never feel better with the drugs; the only way to change how she felt was to use everything she had learned about recovery. Five years later, the woman is still sober.

Carol flushes the pills down the toilet and calls that woman. Carol meets with this woman that evening and recommits to recovery, to the long-term care plan she had been assigned, and to honestly sharing her real feelings with her peers. She recognizes that she has been given the tools necessary to avert a disaster. Carol is no longer a doctor with a shameful secret. She truly wants to stay clean and sober and is now a member of the recovering community.

Cravings, Triggers, and Perseverance

Initial recovery is very difficult. People have powerful cravings, they are repeatedly triggered by reminders of past experiences, and they have to learn to deal with life without the numbing effects of drugs. They face the consequences of the addiction: medical problems, family dysfunction, job problems, financial disasters, and legal problems. These issues are often avoided during active addiction, but after treatment, they must be dealt with.

Early abstinence is a very stressful time, and people in early recovery are extremely vulnerable to the siren call of the addictive drug. Their brains are still altered by the drug, primed to return to that which controlled them. It is not surprising that so many addicts relapse. Treatment that involves active participation over extended periods is the best resource to improve recovery rates.

Medical science is also beginning to provide medications that can promote abstinence, and dramatic new findings will continue to improve these efforts. Anything that will help improve the recovery rate, particularly during the first twelve to eighteen months, will be a boon to the individuals and families affected by addictive disease. Lasting recovery from addictive disease can result in remarkable improvements in people's lives. This is one of the real gifts for the professionals in the addiction field: they get to witness this transformation.

Carol has recommitted to recovery and never again doubts the wisdom in attending to all the activities required of her. She knows it saved her from a disastrous relapse, perhaps even saved her life. She admits the episode at her groups and finds others willing to share similar experiences, most ending up in relapse. She learns that many of the people in her Twelve Step meetings have experienced relapse, some tragic, but she also experiences remarkable support from her peers. She gets phone lists and invitations to social events, and she finds herself attending more meetings to be with new friends.

Carol's cravings slowly begin to fade over the next several months, and work becomes somewhat routine again. She finds herself more involved with her surgical patients, more caring and empathic, as she can sense their fear and vulnerability in a way she hasn't noticed since medical school. She finds support from colleagues who she feared would dismiss her, and re-establishes friendships in the workplace.

Carol begins to lead the life she longed for, a life she is once again proud of, and gradually the shame slips away. She starts skiing and hiking again, activities she had quit within months of starting the Vicodin. Her confidence returns and she starts dating. She works out a system with her ex-husband so she can meet with her children, supervised at first, on a weekly basis. This means more than all the other changes combined. After eighteen months clean and sober, they establish a new custody agreement and Carol is able to bring her children home and be the mother they need and love.

Miracles do occur in recovery, and the damage caused by addiction can be healed. Carol did not choose to become an addict, nor did she choose to undermine her family and her career, but the powerful unbridled nature of this misunderstood disease took away her ability to avoid such calamity. With appropriate treatment, she was given the tools that led to a choice: she could return to drug use and the predictable deterioration or continue the work necessary for personal growth in recovery.

How to Intervene on a
Loved One's Addiction

Robert J. Meyers, Ph.D., and John Gardin, Ph.D.

Ray, returning home from work, walks in the door and finds his wife, Anne, sleeping on the sofa for the third time this week. The sink is full of dirty dishes, and Anne is still in her pajamas. As Ray tries to wake her, she pushes him away and asks to be left alone. Ray finally wakes her up and asks her the same questions he has been asking her for the last several weeks: "Why are you always so tired in the afternoon?" and "What's wrong with you?"

In her usual fashion, Anne shrugs off Ray's questions and with her eyes half-closed tells him in a thick, slightly slurred voice, "I work hard taking care of the house during the day and what's wrong with a little nap?"

Ray has not yet realized that Anne's slurred speech, drowsiness, interrupted sleep patterns, and lethargy are all side effects from abusing the pills her doctor prescribed for her—abuse that is rapidly proceeding to addiction. Anne has been acting oddly for many months, but Ray has rationalized that it is just part of the empty-nest syndrome. Their youngest child started college the previous fall, and for the first time since they were married, they are without any children at home. Both Anne and Ray were very involved in their children's lives, and now, with no kids around, it seems like they have stopped doing everything that used to bring them pleasure—like taking long walks and going to the movies.

They have had a wonderful marriage—Ray would be the first to acknowledge that—but now it all seems to be unraveling. Anne complained about feeling anxious, even before their last child left home, and her physician gave her a prescription to help her relax. Over the past seven months, Anne has been taking more and more of the pills to get the desired feeling. Ray has no clue that Anne is taking up to ten pills a day, although her prescription calls for only two pills a day.

If a Little Is Good, More Is *Not* Better

Anne, like most people who become addicted to prescription medication, started using her medicine just as prescribed by her physician. Initially, the pills didn't seem to help much, so her doctor increased the dose to what he called a "therapeutic level." Medications work differently for different people, and modifying the dose, or finding the therapeutic level, is standard medical practice. Once the physician and Anne got the dosage right, it seemed to help. But for a variety of reasons— some psychological, some biological, some genetic, and many more that we still don't understand—Anne began abusing her prescription medication, taking the pills in increasing amounts. She thought, as many prescription abusers do, "If a little is good, then more is better." Pretty soon, she began to need her pills, and her use moved from abuse to addiction.

Recognizing the signs of drug addiction, or even abuse, is not as easy as it may seem. And even if our loved one is clearly demonstrating signs of addiction, we often don't want to see the signs. Ray has been noticing Anne's slurred speech, drowsiness, interrupted sleep, memory loss, and mental confusion, but he doesn't want to admit that there might be a problem. Why? Because it's scary, and acknowledging a drug problem is one thing, but doing something about that problem is another. For Ray, that would mean having to deal directly with Anne and her problem, for which he is not well-equipped.

The truth is, most loved ones of drug addicts (especially prescription drug addicts) don't know much about drug problems, but they know even less about the options available to intervene for drug problems. Hoping that somehow Anne will see that the pills given to *help* with a problem have now *become* a problem, Ray continues to give Anne the benefit of the doubt again and again.

It's important to note here that prescription drug addiction and prescription drug abuse are very serious medical problems. We do not recommend that anyone abruptly change the amount of medication he or she is taking—even if that person wants to stop abusing pills—without consulting a physician.

Seeing the Forest and the Trees

One day at work, Ray decides to discuss his situation with his old friend George. Ray has known George since college. In those days, Ray and George used to go out drinking together. On occasion, they also used marijuana and other illegal drugs. But after college, Ray got tired of the party scene and focused more on his family and work. George, on the other hand, kept on drinking and partying.

Eventually, George's life began to unravel and he sought treatment for his drug problems. Ray reasoned that because George has maintained several years of recovery from drug problems, he might be a good resource. George suggests that Ray consult a professional, either in the mental health or substance abuse field, because from what Ray is telling him, Anne has a serious drug problem. Initially, Ray is outraged and dismisses the idea. He calls his friend an "AA crazy."

Ray, like so many other concerned family members, refuses to see the forest for the trees and does not want to believe his wife has a problem with prescription medication. It is easier for Ray to tell himself that his wife is just overreacting to the kids leaving or that she is overwhelmed by some other problem. Ray wants the problem to just go away—somehow.

After a few more weeks, with Ray approaching the end of his rope, he begins a cycle of nagging, pleading, and threatening Anne about the changes he is seeing—changes that make his life more uncomfortable and changes that scare him. The more Ray pushes on Anne, the worse things get at home. The tension at home is barely tolerable.

Nagging, Threatening, and Pleading

Nagging, threatening, and pleading are natural reactions to a loved one's drug abuse. Unfortunately, these tactics often only make matters worse. Whatever moments of peace remain in Ray's and Anne's lives are now quickly dissolving. Ray is doing what comes naturally. He has not been trained or educated in how to deal with such a problem. He just wants the problem to go away.

During this time, Ray comes home from work to find Anne lying on the floor in a stupor. She is difficult to wake up, and once awake, she is so disoriented that she cannot remember how she ended up on the floor. Ray, on the verge of panic, wants to call 911, but Anne pleads with him not to. Finally, Ray begins to see that he needs to take matters into his own hands. Even though he is very embarrassed, he decides to talk again to his friend George. George gives him the name of Mr. Jones, a local counselor with a reputation for knowing what to do with drug and alcohol problems.

Anne's reaction to Ray's attempt to call 911 is very typical. Anne may realize, at some level, that she has a problem. But she, like Ray, is scared and doesn't know what to do about it. She only knows, at this point, that taking her pills is the only thing that seems to make her problems go away. And now, on top of the original problem that started it all (her anxiety), she has other problems: a marriage that is unraveling and a need for more medication.

Ray, having run out of options and with nowhere else to turn, makes an appointment to see Mr. Jones. Ray begins the first session by telling Mr. Jones how hopeless he feels his marriage has become, and that he really doesn't know what to do. He also finds himself filled with anger, frustration, and more emotions than he has previously realized.

A New Intervention Model

Mr. Jones, who is well-trained in intervention techniques, allows Ray to vent his emotions before suggesting to Ray a program made for the type of problem he is describing. The program is called CRAFT (Community Reinforcement and Family Training).[1] Mr. Jones tells Ray all about CRAFT, describing it as a science-based intervention model designed to help individuals, like Ray, motivate a drug-affected family member, like Anne, into treatment.

This new intervention model was developed from the belief that family members can and do make important contributions to their loved one's addiction *treatment* and that family members can play a powerful role in getting an addicted loved one into treatment. In fact, the addict in treatment often reports that family pressure or influence is the reason he or she finally sought treatment. Mr. Jones also tells Ray that the CRAFT program will benefit Ray by helping him to become more independent and by reducing his negative emotions, such as depression, anxiety, and anger.

The intervention techniques used in the CRAFT approach have been proven to prompt treatment-resistant drug abusers into treatment 70 percent of the time.[2] In addition to better participation in treatment, the quality of life of the concerned significant others (CSOs) improves greatly. Ray will have a better quality of life after going through the process, whether his loved one enters treatment or not.

Mr. Jones quickly points out that CRAFT uses an overall positive approach and never resorts to confrontation, as do many other approaches. Instead, CRAFT emphasizes learning new skills to cope with old problems. He reassures Ray that Anne is abusing her pills for specific reasons and that once they understand those reasons, they will be able to help her find better ways to cope with her problems without the use of pills.

The Using Map

After sharing the overall goal and structure of CRAFT, Mr. Jones suggested to Ray that they develop a "using map," a three-step process describing in detail the *before, during,* and *after* aspects of Anne's drug using behavior.

First, Ray needs to identify the *before* signs—often called *triggers*—that are associated with Anne's drug use. Mr. Jones compares these triggers to road signs that warn what's ahead. The road signs that let Ray know when Anne is about to use might include moods, thoughts, times, events, and what she says or doesn't say—anything that precedes and is related to Anne's using behavior. Ray begins listing these behaviors during the first session, and he is asked by Mr. Jones to complete the list before his next appointment.

Ray leaves his session and for the first time has some real hope for his marriage. He feels he can give this new approach an opportunity to work. In fact, one of the more notable effects of the CRAFT approach is that loved ones are given hope based on sound research. Over and over again, in multiple clinical trials, CRAFT has proven to engage treatment-resistant drug abusers and addicts into treatment 70 percent of the time. So when Mr. Jones asks Ray to give this approach a try, Mr. Jones knows they have a 70 percent chance that Anne will seek treatment within a couple of months. That fact alone gives Ray real hope, and with that renewed hope, Ray's depression and anxiety begin to shrink.

Also, you will notice that Mr. Jones gave Ray something to do between sessions. Homework is an integral part of the CRAFT approach. CRAFT begins by outlining the context in which substance-abusing behavior occurs, and it teaches the CSO how to use positive reinforcers (rewards) as well as how to let the substance abuser experience the natural consequences of his or her using behavior.

This approach acknowledges that no one has better information about the substance abuser's or addict's behavior patterns than a close family member. With guidance, the CSO can learn how to use this information in a motivational way to increase the chance of the substance abuser or addict agreeing to get the help he or she needs.

A New Focus

During the week between his first and second appointments, Ray gives a lot of thought to what events, thoughts, or moods precede Anne's using. And he is surprised at what he discovers. For one thing, he realizes that he knows a lot more about his wife and her behavior that relates to her use of pills than he originally thought. He also realizes that he is much tenser and hyper-alert than he had realized. It begins to dawn on Ray that by changing *how* he looks at his wife and her using, and *what* he looks at, his mood begins to change too—and for the better.

CSOs are often surprised by what they find out when they stop focusing on how to stop their loved one, from using, stop trying to control their loved one, and start focusing on what their loved one is actually doing. Often this exercise allows the CSO to look at the loved one's use through different eyes— eyes not of judgment or disgust or frustration, but eyes with just a glimmer of understanding, eyes that are looking for solutions.

This new focus allows Ray to connect the dots related to Anne's use of pills. It also gives him permission to see what he has not wanted to see. Remember, we talked about how loved ones don't want to see what they don't know how to fix? Now that Ray has been given just the start of a process that holds out the hope of "fixing" what's wrong, he is able to look more clearly and carefully at what's going on in Anne's life. What he's about to find out is that he is often able to predict whether Anne will use her pills or not, based on what's going on in Anne's life. He also discovers that a trigger may or may not result in Anne using her pills. Just as an exit sign on the freeway signals an exit ahead, it doesn't mean you have to take it.

The Trigger List

At his second session, Ray is excited to share with Mr. Jones what he learned about Anne's using. Ray actually feels relieved in sharing his homework assignments. The trigger list looks like this:

ANNE'S TRIGGERS

➡ when she has no plans; an "empty" day

➡ when she starts complaining about being "uptight" or "nervous"

➡ after our daughter calls from college

➡ when she is very quiet and withdrawn

➡ when she can't seem to sit still

Having Ray carefully and thoughtfully examine Anne's using behavior is an important first step toward intervening or helping change that behavior. First of all, Anne's using behavior begins to make sense to Ray. It's no longer a mystical process tied to unseen and unknown causes over which he or she may or may not have control. Instead, Ray now can get a handle on what may be some of Anne's reasons for using too many pills and how the pills help her cope with her demons. This perspective not only sets the stage for intervention tactics but also helps to move Ray from his anger and frustration into a more constructive problem-solving mode. That doesn't mean that Ray won't still have negative feelings to work through, but it does mean that he now has a positive focus as well. And in time, he will become more positive and understanding and less accusatory.

Using Signs

Mr. Jones tells Ray that this is a great start, and that knowing these triggers will help them eventually help Anne. But he reminds Ray that the entire "using map" will need to be completed, and this is only the first of three parts. The second part involves how Ray knows when Anne is using. Mr. Jones tells Ray that often the signs of drug abuse and addiction are obvious—like when Anne was in a stupor on the floor. But other times the signs might not be so obvious.

Mr. Jones asks Ray to recall how Anne acts when she is using—not the passed-out-on-the-floor using, but the kind of using that might lead to more subtle signs. Ray comes up blank, so Mr. Jones gives him some examples: maybe Anne's voice becomes louder or softer; maybe she talks slower or faster; maybe her physical appearance changes in some way; perhaps her behavior is affected (she is less responsive or over-responsive). The examples help Ray to look for the small changes that he has been aware of for some time but has chosen to ignore.

With Mr. Jones's help, Ray identifies the following as signs that Anne might be using (and, of course, abusing) her pills:

ANNE'S USING SIGNS (BEHAVIORS)

- she becomes less talkative—answering questions with simple, short responses
- she is less concerned about her looks, so that her makeup is messed up or her hair is unkempt
- she eats less (she usually has a good appetite)
- she doesn't answer the phone
- she doesn't come to bed with me, but stays up and sleeps on the sofa

As stated earlier, some signs of using are easy to see while some are more subtle. Helping Ray get clear on these signs will better enable him to know when Anne has been using and when she hasn't been using. Often, once a CSO has completed this section of the map, he or she comes to realize that the loved one is using either more or less than the CSO had at first believed. Studies have shown, however, that a CSO's report of a loved one's use is usually very accurate. Later, as actual intervention steps are created to be used by Ray, it will be crucial that he has completed this part of the map.

Mr. Jones explains that even though it might have been uncomfortable to identify these behaviors, it is a very important step, and he tells Ray that he has done a great job. Mr. Jones constantly uses positive reinforcement with Ray. This serves to increase Ray's compliance and involvement and also models for Ray how to use positive reinforcement—a powerful tool that plays a pivotal role in the CRAFT approach.

Consequences of Using

Mr. Jones asks Ray if he is ready for the third part of mapping Anne's using behavior: identifying the consequences of her using. Ray is starting to get the hang of this and is ready to proceed. Mr. Jones suggests that Ray begin by thinking about all of the consequences of Anne's use—what happens after she uses. Mr. Jones is quick to point out that although most of these consequences would most certainly be negative, there might also be positive consequences to her use as well. Ray is able to identify the following consequences:

ANNE'S USING CONSEQUENCES

➡ we argue about her using

➡ she spends less time with her friends

➟ she misses phone calls from our daughter

➟ we have next to no sex life

➟ she doesn't do her share of the housework

Mr. Jones tells Ray that this is an excellent start, and that he wonders whether Ray might also experience some payoff as a result of Anne's using. Initially, Ray is offended at the question and asks, "How could I possibly get anything positive out of her use?" But with gentle prodding, Ray admits that Anne's using has had some positive aspects to it. Examples are as follows:

- When Anne is using, I don't have to listen to her go on and on about a subject I have no interest in, such as a television show she saw on the design channel.

- Her using gives me an excuse to spend more time in the garage working on projects rather than be with her.

- When she is subdued, I can do anything I want to do.

A Loved One's Using Map

If you are living with someone whom you suspect is addicted to or abusing pills, you can use the following chart to begin mapping out the using patterns of your loved one, just as Ray did with his therapist. Use the chart on the next page to help you.

A Loved One's Using Map

Triggers for a Loved One's Use of Drugs or Alcohol

- _____
- _____
- _____
- _____
- _____

Signs that Your Loved One Has Been Using

- _____
- _____
- _____
- _____
- _____

Consequences of a Loved One's Use

- _____
- _____
- _____
- _____
- _____

A Clear Picture

Getting a clear picture of what happens after Anne uses is an important piece in the map of her using behavior. Ray will now, with Mr. Jones's help, be able to lay out a clear picture of the *before, during,* and *after* of Anne's using.

Here's the way it's looking so far: Anne's life has lots of holes in it, especially since her youngest daughter left for college. With more empty time on her hands, she probably spends more time thinking about how lonely she is, which only makes her lonelier. To ease the pain of loneliness and the anxiety that comes with it, she takes a pill to help her relax— and forget. But as she relaxes and forgets, she becomes less and less interactive with Ray, the main source of support in her life at this time. She also withdraws from others in her life, and when she gets a call from her daughter, whom she misses terribly, Anne won't talk to her because she doesn't feel well. Anne is getting less and less of what she really wants. To Ray's great dismay, she also tends to let herself go when using, and she doesn't keep up the house like she used to. This annoys Ray, so he badgers her at night, resulting in repeated arguments. They often do not even sleep together, and if they do, there is never sex.

Toward the end of the second session, Mr. Jones tells Ray that their using map is just about complete. The only piece left is to determine a "baseline" of current pattern of use. Mr. Jones explains that determining the pattern of Anne's use will accomplish two things:

- it will complete the map, or picture, of Anne's use
- it will allow Ray to notice changes in Anne's use as they occur

So Mr. Jones asks Ray to think about his best estimate of how many pills Anne takes and how often she takes them. Of course, Ray can't be with Anne every minute of every day, so Mr. Jones suggests that he just go with his instincts, making the best guess he can. Ray tells Mr. Jones how many pills he thinks Anne is taking each day of the week, and when he thinks she is taking them.

At the end of this session, Ray is exhausted but encouraged that they have accomplished so much. Mr. Jones suggests that Ray take everything that they have discussed—the before, during, and after of Anne's use—and draw out on a sheet of paper a map of how things move from "before" through "during" to "after" with one or two of Anne's most common triggers.

He asks Ray to get as specific as he can in describing what happens, including answering the following: Is she alone when she is taking her pills? What is she doing? Where is she? When is she taking her pills? Why is she taking her pills? Although willing to do this assignment, Ray questions Mr. Jones about how much longer this CRAFT therapy thing will take. He's not sure he can put up with Anne's using much longer. Timing is everything, and Mr. Jones knows that he should not let Ray start any new "intervention" process until he is prepared.

Staying with the Plan

It has taken two sessions to get to the place where the basic details—the map of Anne's using behaviors—have been identified. This is not an easy or comfortable process. Often, CSOs come to this point and feel as overwhelmed as they were when they first came into counseling. Somehow, speaking the truth about Anne makes intervening even more urgent in Ray's mind. Not surprisingly, Ray, like most CSOs, wants results immediately. He has been living with Anne's using—and all the uncomfortable and scary changes associated with that using—for months. Many CSOs have been living with these types of problems for years, or even decades, and they want something to change *now*. So Ray's impatience is neither unusual nor unwarranted.

Mr. Jones reminds Ray that Anne's using behaviors will not change without intervening, and that by taking this time to explore and describe her use, they have laid the foundation for an effective intervention, one that will lead to Anne entering treatment. Mr. Jones points out that documenting her using behaviors is part of the process and things will begin to move at a faster pace. Now they need to fashion an intervention designed specifically to help change Anne's using behavior. He reminds Ray that he needs to stick to the plan and see what happens. With hard work, they have a great chance that within a couple of weeks, Anne will be ready to seek treatment. Ray agrees to continue working the CRAFT program. He agrees to come back next week with a couple of diagrams of Anne's using behaviors.

When Ray returns the following week for his third session, he has his homework, and he reports that Anne is, inexplicably, using less. He insists that he hasn't changed anything, other than to stop harassing her so much. When asked why he has stopped harassing her, he replies that he was just too busy observing what's going on to get upset by it. He has also been told by Mr. Jones that nagging, pleading, and complaining have not worked in the past, and he is very sure they won't work now.

Subtle Change

The CRAFT approach is based on cognitive-behavioral principles that have been shown to be highly effective. We also know that whenever we change anything in a system, the system makes adjustments to that change. Ray, following instructions from Mr. Jones, has adopted a new position with Anne, one of trying to understand rather than trying to control, and Anne has now responded. With less pressure from Ray to stop using her pills, she has picked up on the cue and started to use less. It is often true that the harder we push someone, the harder they resist that push or even push back. One of the truly powerful outcomes observed in an alcohol study of CRAFT was that the alcohol-dependent individual reduced his or her drinking by 50 percent before he or she ever entered treatment.[3] The same may be said for prescription medication abusers and addicts.

Ray then gives Mr. Jones the following description of a typical argument and how it has not been successful in getting Anne to cut down on her pill use.

> I come home and find Anne frazzled ➡ I start to tell her about my day, hoping to distract her ➡ Anne doesn't respond, but instead says she needs to "take something" ➡ I tell her that she doesn't need to take anything ➡ She tells me I don't understand ➡ I tell her that she just needs to "get over it" ➡ She takes her pill ➡ I begin harassing her for taking her pill ➡ We start arguing ➡ She goes to our bedroom and shuts the door ➡ I go out to the garage

Ray reports that he still doesn't see how this particular situation could possibly turn out any other way. With the help of Mr. Jones, however, he starts exploring alternative ways of interacting with Anne in this situation that might result in a different outcome. Ray starts to see that the power he has in the relationship is not a function of what he can *control*, but of how he *responds* to Anne. He acknowledges that his initial response is based on his belief that, after all, she's been home all day doing nothing, while he's been out there slaying dragons.

Ray has no patience for her situation, and so he reacts by turning the focus on himself, which, of course, doesn't work. Once he understands that what he has been doing doesn't work, he is willing to consider other options. After all, the ultimate goal is to positively affect Anne's use, and by reminding Ray of this goal, Mr. Jones is able to help him move forward with creative alternatives.

Mr. Jones reminds Ray of Anne's triggers, the overall picture of her using, and the central role that loneliness appears to play in her life. He asks Ray what he thinks he might do to help Anne feel less lonely. As Ray thinks about it, he is able to write out another map—one that he thinks might just work. The parts below in parentheses are what he used to do; the parts in bold are what he is now going to do.

> I come home and find Anne frazzled ➠ (I start to tell her about my day, hoping to distract her) **Instead of ignoring how she is feeling, I invite her to sit down on the floor in front of me while I sit on the sofa so I can give her a neck massage** ➠ (Anne doesn't respond, but instead says she needs to "take something") **She begins to share how she is feeling** ➠ (I tell her that she doesn't need to take anything) **I let her know that I care about her and how she is feeling and suggest that we fix dinner together like we used to when we were first married** ➠ (She tells me I don't understand) **We have a good time fixing dinner** ➠ (I tell her that she just needs to "get

over it" ➡ She takes her pill ➡ I begin harassing her for taking her pill ➡ We start arguing ➡ She goes to our bedroom and shuts the door ➡ I go out to the garage) ➡ **We spend the evening together listening to music or watching TV and go to bed together**

As demonstrated, this new way of communicating in a positive way is much more effective. Since Ray knew that a trigger for Anne was loneliness, he just gave her some much-desired attention. Ray didn't need to discuss how sad Anne was that their daughter was gone (although that might be appropriate too) or how isolated she had become. He merely met an unmet need that had become a trigger for Anne.

Backup Plans

Mr. Jones congratulates Ray on coming up with what looks like a great plan. He then brainstorms with Ray about how this plan might go awry, and what backup plans he might need.

Life doesn't always go as planned. Although what Ray has outlined looks good, there are many points at which things could take a turn for the worse. Looking for potential problems ahead of time will help to refine Ray's plan. Also, having a backup plan is important. If something goes wrong, Ray won't be caught flat-footed. He'll have another course of action.

Ray has decided on giving Anne a neck massage as a primary plan. If she is not in the mood for this, he is ready to suggest that they go for a walk. That's something that they used to do together, and he knows that Anne also likes taking walks—or she used to like taking walks. And another backup plan is that if she doesn't want to cook dinner together, he'll offer to take them out to dinner.

Ray can't, of course, cover every possibility. But a good plan is one that is well thought out. It's also important that the plan of action not involve things that have failed in the past. If Anne really doesn't like neck massages, then suggesting a neck massage would not be a good idea. If walking together had resulted in battles over who was walking too fast or too slow in the past, then walking would not be a good idea either.

Mr. Jones congratulates Ray on setting up a very good plan and is optimistic about it turning out well. "But what if in the middle of all this Anne decides to take a pill?" Mr. Jones asks. How should Ray react? Ray is instructed to give this scenario some thought. Ray admits that if that happens he's stumped. It would seem that if Anne decides to take a pill during the process, the whole plan has failed. The therapist points out that even if she does take a pill, he can respond in a way that will not make the situation worse. He suggests that Ray might say something like "You know, honey, that I love you and would be happy to give you a neck massage, but after you've taken one of those pills, you're just not yourself, so I think I'll just go upstairs and read for a while."

Ray is learning a new approach, one that makes it more likely that Anne will decrease her using behavior and increase her sober or non-using behavior. Part of the CRAFT model is always to keep communication positive. One of the reasons we use the map is to help establish positive solutions. Introducing behaviors that have been traditionally positive events—like neck massages or walks or cooking together—should result in increased non-using behavior simply because the desired result—being more relaxed and less anxious—can be achieved without using a pill. Anne must learn this lesson, and Ray is helping her to start that process.

Sometimes, however, it's also necessary to remove something that the addict wants in order to get less using behavior. We know Anne is lonely, and in the past, Anne and Ray have spent many hours of quality time together. So when Ray leaves the room after explaining to Anne that she is just not herself when she is choosing to use, he increases the likelihood of her not using in the future, if the company of Ray is something that she really wants.

Working the Plan

Armed with this new plan of action, Ray is very optimistic about the coming week. Sure enough, within a day or two, he has his opportunity to try his plan. As he walks in the door, he notices that Anne seems anxious and on edge. He sticks to his plan, and instead of ignoring her or nagging at her, he invites her to sit at his feet in front of the sofa while he gives her a neck massage. To his surprise, Anne stops dead in her tracks, thanks him, and tells him that she would love a neck massage, but she just wants to take a pill first.

Ray becomes angry and is tempted to fall back into the old path, but he sticks to the plan. Ray says, "Honey, I really would like to give you a neck massage and spend the evening with you, but you're just not the same when you take a pill, so if you're going to take a pill, I'm going to go upstairs and read for a while. Oh, and I love you." Anne once again seems to freeze in her tracks. She had expected Ray to argue with her or to yell at her just like he has done in the past. She was expecting almost anything but the kind, loving words that she is hearing. Even so, she really feels like she needs that pill, and so she goes to the bathroom to find her bottle of pills. Ray goes upstairs to read.

The next night when Ray comes home, Anne is once again pretty wound up. According to his plan, Ray doesn't give up easily and once again offers to give Anne a neck massage. This time, Anne not only thanks him for the offer, but actually gives in and allows him to give her a massage without taking a pill. The rest of the evening goes as planned, and for the first time in months, they go to bed together without a wall of tension and pain between them.

At his next session, Ray is very excited to share with Mr. Jones how the week had gone with Anne, and Mr. Jones is genuinely happy that Ray had such a positive experience. He explains to Ray that this is a good start and that continuing with the map and working on additional new behaviors should continue to build from here. He also suggests to Ray that he give some thought to what he would like his relationship with Anne to look like beyond her not abusing her pills.

Mr. Jones explains to Ray that Anne's using behavior has now created an opportunity to remake their relationship into more of what he would really like it to be. More of what they both would like it to be. So he challenges Ray to examine carefully what might be missing and to think about what their perfect relationship might look like. He also tells Ray to remember the initial attraction and other good things of their relationship that brought them together in the first place. What kinds of activities and events did they used to enjoy? Who were the people they spent time with?

The Seeds of Restoration

It is difficult to reach a destination if you don't know where you're going. For Ray to move from merely helping Anne to stop her addiction to pills to improving the quality of their lives together will take some careful thought and consideration.

This exercise allows Ray to get in touch with what had been lost in their relationship and to lay the foundation for reclaiming it. It is amazing how the seeds for restoration are often found in what at first looks like destruction.

Ray comes up with a description of his perfect relationship with Anne and shares it with Mr. Jones:

> I would like Anne and me to start doing more things like we used to. We used to ride our bikes every Saturday along the river, and I'd like to do that again. I'd like us to go out to dinner and to the movies once or twice a week. I'd like to have Barry and Jean over. They're our closest friends, but we stopped seeing them quite awhile ago when Anne's behavior became so unpredictable. I'd like for us to play cards with our friends again. I'd like for us to be able to spend time talking about our future together now that the kids are gone. I'd like us to start attending church again.

As Ray shares his desires for his relationship with Anne, it is obvious to Mr. Jones that these things are very important to Ray. At points, Ray smiles broadly as he remembers how it used to be with Anne.

The kind of emotional energy revealed by Ray is crucial to fuel the process of change. Ray must remember that things don't change overnight and that this process is often a long and bumpy road. His initial gains must sustain and carry him through the occasional disappointment. Change takes time, and the persistence and perseverance necessary is fed by how rewarding the final goal of a comfortable and happy life with Anne, without the use of drugs, will be.

Remaking the Relationship

Mr. Jones then helps Ray with the next step: designing a plan for the coming week. The goal is to begin to work on the relationship with Anne that Ray has described. Given that Anne's behavior is not entirely predictable, Mr. Jones suggests that Ray start with a behavior that is on the safe side and very likely to have a positive outcome. Ray decides to ask Anne to go to the movies or on a bike ride. The therapist reminds Ray that it is important that he move slowly as not to overwhelm Anne with too many new activities. And he reminds Ray that he should only invite Anne to participate if she is not abusing her pills.

Mr. Jones also reminds Ray that his role in the remaking of this relationship is a key element, so it is essential that Ray also take proper care of himself. Mr. Jones compares Ray's position to that of a rescuer of a drowning swimmer: unless the rescuer is a very good swimmer and knows what to do, jumping in to save the person drowning will probably result in them both going down. So what does Ray need to do to take care of himself? What activities has he given up that used to bring him satisfaction or a sense of well-being? What other relationships has he let go of in order to take care of Anne?

Mr. Jones reminds Ray that part of their goal in the CRAFT program is to help Ray enjoy his life. Although Ray has set many goals that involve Anne, it is also important to set some personal goals around helping Ray feel better about himself without Anne being involved. Ray is told to think of pleasurable activities in three general areas:

1. things that he can do to feel better that are free and instantaneous

2. things that he can do to feel better that involve a minimal amount of money and time

3. things that he can do to feel better that involve moderate to significant amounts of money and time

Ray comes up with this list of activities:

1. free and/or quick activities: give myself compliments, pray more often

2. low-cost and/or minimal time activities: call a friend, go to church, take a walk by myself

3. moderate cost or moderate time activities: go to the gym, go to the movies with a friend

Mr. Jones then suggests that Ray make time during the coming week for some of these activities.

Ray, like most loved ones of those abusing pills, alcohol, or other drugs, has constricted his life to compensate for the strain and embarrassment he has been experiencing. It is very important that he begin to enjoy some social and recreational times that he has eliminated from his life due to Anne's addiction. With this new balance, Ray will have more energy to invest in his relationship and in the entire CRAFT process.

During the week after his fourth session, Ray is amazed at how much more optimistic he feels. He goes to the gym, where he hasn't been in months, and meets a friend for a cup of coffee. He finds himself feeling much more in control and is better able to interact positively with Anne, spending more time with her when she is not abusing her pills.

Ray also does not react negatively when Anne is using her pills. He notices that she is making an effort to use pills less often. He now writes down in a log all the times he feels Anne is abusing drugs, and the episodes seem to be diminishing.

When Ray arrives for his next session, he describes how

much better Anne is doing, and how much better he feels as well. He proudly reports that he worked out twice in the last week, called a friend, attended church, and feels better. He still finds himself taking care of Anne when she is abusing her pills, though, such as making dinner for them both and then keeping hers warm until she is with it enough to eat it.

Enabling

Mr. Jones points out that by making and warming Anne's dinner for her, Ray is *enabling* her. The therapist explains that enabling means consciously or unconsciously helping a loved one maintain negative drug-using behavior. Ray objects, stating that it's important that she eat, and if he doesn't make her dinner and keep it warm, she will miss a meal. On top of that, she'll get mad and accuse him of not caring about her.

One of the more difficult tasks for loved ones of a drug abuser to learn is that some of what they do actually helps the abuser continue the abusing behavior. Ray's intentions are good, but his actions only serve to allow Anne's abuse to proceed without her experiencing some of the natural negative consequences of her abuse. Another important aspect of CRAFT is helping loved ones understand that a huge factor in learning to change behavior is the experience of those natural negative consequences. Because Ray has taken care of Anne when she is using (making sure that she eats), Anne isn't experiencing one of the negative effects, or consequences, of her use.

Mr. Jones explains to Ray the concept of natural negative consequences, and that by not allowing Anne to experience the natural negative consequence of her drug abuse, he is actually rewarding her abuse. In other words, from Anne's perspective, when she is abusing her pills and Ray makes sure she still eats, there's no downside to her abuse. As long as Ray is taking care of her, why would she want to stop abusing her pills? Ray is insistent that, even though he makes and warms her meals, he always tells her off in the process, and surely that can't feel good to Anne, so how is that enabling? Mr. Jones points out, "It must not feel that bad to her because it hasn't affected her pill abuse yet, has it?"

Why Nagging Doesn't Work

Ray has to admit that all the warm meals accompanied by his nagging have had no affect at all. It is business as usual. Mr. Jones suggests that instead of making and warming the meals, Ray merely leave the food in the refrigerator. He also suggests that Ray give up entirely nagging or trying to reason with Anne when she is under the influence of drugs. Nagging hasn't had any noticeable effect on Anne's use so far, so why keep doing the same thing over and over if it is not working?

Initially, Ray resists the term *nagging*. He defends what he says to Anne, stating, "I don't really nag at her as much as let her know how her pill abuse is really messing with our lives." Mr. Jones tells Ray that he understands how it doesn't seem like nagging to Ray, but he asks Ray how he thinks Anne views it. Ray has to admit that no matter how carefully he words it, she says he is nagging her.

Mr. Jones suggests that instead of telling Anne about what *she is doing* that he doesn't approve of, he can tell her about what *he is feeling*. Ray looks blank at this point. The only feeling he is able to identify is feeling really ticked off. But as he and Mr. Jones talk, Ray comes to realize that he is feeling angry, hurt, and lonely, and that he truly misses his wife and the relationship that he and Anne once enjoyed.

Mr. Jones works with Ray to come up with ways of expressing his feelings to Anne. After some coaching, Ray comes up with the statement "I really miss having dinner with you but it's too uncomfortable for me to eat with you when you're not yourself. I'll leave your food in the fridge if I feel that I can't handle eating with you."

Mr. Jones also suggests that Ray have a conversation with Anne when she is not using about how much he misses eating with her. Mr. Jones and Ray spend some time role-playing the situation so Ray will be comfortable with how to talk to Anne in a positive and supportive way. Ray agrees that when he feels that she has been abusing her pills, he will just leave her food in the fridge for her to eat later.

Ray agrees to try this new strategy next week. Mr. Jones also asks Ray to make a list of all the ways he has attempted to get Anne to stop abusing her pills in the past. He explains to Ray that looking carefully at what has not worked will help them avoid making the same mistakes over and over. If something has not worked in the past, it probably won't work now either.

During the following week, Ray nags Anne less and engages in upbeat conversation every opportunity he gets. He finds himself feeling less controlled by Anne's pill abuse. He also feels that he is having more of a positive affect on her using behaviors. He notices how much better he is feeling since he has started working out, praying more, and interacting with old friends. Anne is still abusing her pills, but it seems to him that she continues to use them less.

Communication Tips

In their sixth session, Mr. Jones listens to Ray as he describes the preceding week. He then tells Ray that he would like to share some communication principles with him. He tells Ray that whenever relationships come upon hard times, whether it's related to drug addiction or not, certain changes are very predictable. To help partners use good communication skills, one must (1) be **P**ositive, (2) begin with an **"I"** statement, (3) use **U**nderstanding, and (4) show a willingness to **S**hare responsibility. Mr. Jones points out that an easy way to remember these changes is by the acronym PIUS.

As a relationship becomes more stress-filled, communications are usually filled with negative comments and focus almost entirely on negative events. Partners stop talking about themselves (using "I" statements) and talk more about the other person (using "you" statements). Because the relationship has deteriorated, there is usually very little understanding and much more judging. And there is definitely a tendency to blame and criticize as opposed to sharing any responsibility. All of these traits only serve to further erode a relationship in trouble.

On the other hand, using PIUS communication can help the healing begin. By using PIUS, your loved one will feel less attacked. If your loved one is feeling less attacked, he or she is much less likely to attack back.

Mr. Jones explains the first principle of PIUS (using positive statements) by giving Ray some examples of negative statements:

- The house is always a mess when I come home.
- We never have any fun together anymore.
- I'm tired of you just feeling sorry for yourself.
- I can't stand being around you when you're using those pills.
- I can't talk to you anymore.
- I hate it when you look so out of it.

He then asks Ray to try saying these things in a positive way. Ray struggles, but with Mr. Jones's help, Ray comes up with these positive statements:

- I know keeping the house up is a pain—but I sure appreciate it when it's picked up.
- I miss having fun with you.
- You look pretty down.
- I love being with you when you're not using those pills.
- I miss the long conversations by the fireplace that we used to have, but I don't feel comfortable talking with you after you've taken your pills.
- I remember the twinkle in your eye when I would come home, and now I miss it.

As Ray thought about it, saying things in a positive way makes a lot of sense and often involves using "I" statements—the second part of PIUS. Mr. Jones explains that someone hurling a verbal attack beginning with the word *you* starts most arguments. Ray understands that replacing "you" with "I" will have the effect of telling Anne what he feels or wants—not what she is doing wrong. He correctly figures that that will head off more than a few living-room tugs-of-war.

The third part of PIUS—understanding statements—also makes good sense to Ray. He sees how adding "I know you don't feel like having fun right now" to "I miss having fun with you" will go a long way to show Anne that he really understands how she is feeling. If she feels that he understands her better or that he is even trying to understand her, then she will have less of a need to defend herself. Less defensiveness equals better communication.

Mr. Jones tells Ray that the fourth part of PIUS—offering

to share the responsibility—may sound a little upside down and backward. After all, Ray has been feeling much less entangled with Anne, and that has felt good. But Mr. Jones reminds Ray that the reality is that they *are* entangled. While Ray is absolutely not responsible for Anne's prescription pill addiction, and also does not need to take responsibility for everything that's not working in their relationship, his behavior does affect hers and vice versa. When Mr. Jones explains it that way, it makes more sense for Ray to offer help and assistance to Anne. Adding "I know that I haven't been very understanding lately, and that you probably think I don't care anymore, but I do" to "I miss you" sounds like something to which Anne would respond positively.

Look into Treatment Options

Armed with his new communication skills, Ray is sent home to try them out. But before the end of the session, Mr. Jones explains to Ray that it is important to have options for treatment available when Anne decides she needs help. From what Ray has described to him, Mr. Jones tells Ray about an outpatient program in town that he has worked with in the past. He gives Ray the phone number and suggests that Ray contact the program to see what he thinks about its approach. Mr. Jones suggests that if the program is to Ray's liking, he will need to be prepared to present the option of this program to Anne at just the right time and in just the right way. As they have done so many times before, Mr. Jones leads Ray in some role plays about how he might present the option of treatment to Anne at an opportune time.

That week at home is not all a bed of roses. Ray finds himself criticizing Anne one night after work, and they have one of their worst arguments. The next day, Ray is absolutely committed to not react to Anne the same way, and he comes home ready to use his new skills. As soon as he enters the house, he notices that Anne looks upset. He isn't sure whether she has been using her pills or not, but he starts right in with "Honey, I'm sorry for jumping all over you last night. I just get so worried. I love you and want things to work out and will do anything to help."

Anne bursts into tears and tells him she is scared and doesn't know what to do. She says she is tired of the way her life is going. It is the first time that Anne has admitted to Ray that she knows something is wrong. Ray reassures her that they will figure it out together, but that they might need some help. He tells her that he has the name of a program in town that he thinks might be able to help. She seems receptive, and he holds her for most of the night.

Ray finally tells her that he has been going to therapy and that he feels it is helping him. He then asks her if she would like to join him and attend a therapy session with him. He tells her, "I really love you and I want to work on our relationship. I want our life to be fun and for us to enjoy each other. Please come to just one therapy session and see what happens." Anne agrees to go to one therapy session, for the sake of their relationship.

CRAFT does not always work the same for everyone. It is an individualized treatment that has clear procedures and methods. CRAFT has shown that seven out of ten people who use this method have succeeded in getting a loved one into treatment. We all know that this is just the first step, but it's a big step and can lead to healing, restoration, and long-term success.

The CRAFT approach is much more involved than can possibly be described in a single chapter. Fortunately, Robert

Meyers and Brenda Wolfe have written a book designed to be used as a CRAFT self-help manual.[4] If you love an addict who won't get help, don't give up—buy the book and use it. Find a counselor who has been trained in CRAFT or who is willing to provide you with support as you work through the book. Keep in mind that the CRAFT approach is not for directly treating the addict—only for getting the addict to accept treatment from a trained professional.

OxyContin Addiction

A NEW DRUG, BUT AN OLD PROBLEM

William White, M.A.

The recent media attention generated by OxyContin is only the latest chapter in America's long history of addiction to medically prescribed narcotics and non-narcotic painkillers. In this chapter, we will explore drugs (from alcohol and tobacco to narcotics and cocaine), both patent and prescription, that were used for legitimate medical purposes but had unexpected consequences, including addiction. My intent is neither to castigate all drugs whose excessive or prolonged use can produce substance use disorders, nor indict the drug companies that manufacture them, the physicians who prescribe them, and the pharmacists who distribute them. Many of the drugs discussed here have provided a needed balm to millions. My intent is rather to underscore the shadow side of the long history of the use of psychoactive drugs within American medicine. The goal is to sit at history's feet and see what lessons are offered us on this problem.

OxyContin was introduced into American medicine as a Schedule II prescribed narcotic in December 1995. Its primary active ingredient, oxycodone, has been an ingredient of more than fifty prescribed pain medications (Percodan and Percocet, for example) since the 1960s. OxyContin is distinguished by a high dosage of oxycodone that is time-released. It is this quality that made it an ideal drug in the management of severe pain related to conditions ranging from back injury to cancer. For many patients suffering from severe chronic pain, OxyContin seemed God-sent. Its effectiveness as a painkiller contributed to its rapid popularity.

Reports of OxyContin misuse and addiction increased dramatically in 2002 and 2003. Obtained through forged prescriptions, unscrupulous physicians and pharmacists, theft, and a growing black market, the pills were crushed and snorted or injected to obtain a heroin-like effect. The drug became known as "hillbilly heroin" due to its popularity in economically depressed rural communities such as those found in Appalachia.[1] Alarm over OxyContin addiction was triggered by increased reports of OxyContin-related deaths, emergency room admissions, and addiction treatment admissions.

Complicating the increase in OxyContin use was a parallel increase in the misuse of other narcotic medications, particularly those containing hydrocodone and acetaminophen (Vicodin, Lortab), hydrocodone and aspirin (Lortab ASA), and hydrocodone and ibuprofen (Vicoprofen). Media attention related to celebrity use of drugs containing oxycodone and hydrocodone peaked in 2003, but this was only the tip of the iceberg; this trend is indicated by the fact that the number of people admitted to treatment in the United States for dependence on prescription painkillers doubled between 1992 and 2002.[2]

While this book focuses on a particular category of drugs—prescription narcotics—and a particular drug—OxyContin—that are generating considerable alarm in many communities, this book might also serve as a case study of drugs whose great benefit is stained by their unforeseen potential for misuse and dependence. Preventing and managing this potential in existing and new drugs will require informed leaders and an informed citizenry.

This chapter explores the fascinating history of such drugs, and tries to extract principles for predicting, preventing, and managing what today is referred to as "prescription drug dependence." Our focus will be on two phenomena:

- substance use disorders that emerged out of a process of medical treatment, sometimes referred to as iatrogenic (physician-caused) addiction

- the transition of the manufacture and distribution of psychoactive drugs from legitimate medical channels to illicit drug markets

Patent and Prescription Medicines

Historically, America's legal drugs have come from several sources: 1) herbal home remedies; 2) "ethical" drug companies that manufacture, advertise, and distribute prescription drugs to doctors, hospitals, and pharmacies; and 3) "proprietary" or "patent" drug companies that sell over-the-counter drugs directly to the American public.[3] Psychoactive drugs—including alcohol, opium, morphine, and cocaine—have been staples of the prescription drug and proprietary drug industries, but it was as patent "nostrums" and "secret remedies" that these substances were most widely distributed to American citizens during the eighteenth and nineteenth centuries.

The patent medicine industry reached its peak level of profit and visibility between 1870 and 1930. The value of the "proprietary medicine" industry, as it called itself, rose from $3.5 million in 1859 to $74.5 million in 1903.[4] During this period, the traveling medicine show and the patent medicine catalog were forms of entertainment and the primary source of health care for many Americans. In the late nineteenth and early twentieth centuries, public health reformers championed laws that required truthful labeling of the ingredients of over-the-counter medicines and made physicians and pharmacists the gatekeepers for drugs that had addiction potential.

Tobacco in Medicine

It may shock today's reader to discover that tobacco was once widely used as a medicine. Tobacco was introduced into European medicine in the sixteenth century by the Spanish physician Nicolas de Monardes as a cure for syphilis. In native and colonial America, tobacco was used to treat a broad spectrum of disorders. Tobacco ashes, leaves, and oils were applied to the skin and used to clean teeth. Tobacco juice was applied topically to treat ear and eye infections. Medicines made from the juice of boiled tobacco were given orally. Physicians inserted tobacco snuff into their patients' noses and blew smoke into their patients' mouths to reach their internal organs. Tobacco enemas were given in cases of intestinal disorder, and vaginal injections of tobacco were used to treat gynecological disorders.[5]

The first challenge to the use of tobacco in medicine came in 1798 when America's most prominent physician, Dr. Benjamin Rush, published his essay "Observations upon the Influence of the Habitual Use of Tobacco upon Health, Morals, and Property." Rush attacked the social and medical use of tobacco, noting that, among other problems, it led to excessive drinking.[6]

The beginning of the end of tobacco's use in medicine came in 1828, when two Frenchmen, Heinrich Posselt and

Ludwig Reimann, isolated its primary ingredient. They christened this ingredient "nicotine" after Jean Nicot, the French ambassador to Portugal who had championed the use of tobacco as a medicine. The isolation of nicotine made possible the studies that would eventually document the toxic and addictive properties of nicotine-rich tobacco. Although the medical use of tobacco faded in the mid-1800s, it was more than a century before the devastating effects of tobacco were fully recognized.[7]

Alcohol as Medicine

American home remedies have long contained alcohol, and the presence of alcohol in patent and prescribed medicines increased through the nineteenth century. People who would never consider entering a saloon regularly took alcohol-laced "medicines"—often without knowledge of alcohol's presence. Where alcohol was outlawed as a beverage, the appetite for alcoholic stimulation could be satisfied by high-proof bitters—all in the name of health![8]

Some of the most popular alcohol-laced patent medicines during the nineteenth and early twentieth centuries, and their alcoholic content, included Richardson's Sherry Wine Bitters (47.5 percent), Hostetter's Stomach Bitters (44.3 percent), Parker's Tonic (41.6 percent), Dr. Hartman's Peruna (28.5 percent), Sarsaparilla (26 percent), Lydia Pinkham's Vegetable Compound (21 percent), Hood's Sarsaparilla (18.8 percent), Luther's Temperance Bitters (16.6 percent), and Dr. Kilmer's Swamproot (8.5 percent).[9] Products known as "temperance drinks," but secretly laced with alcohol, such as Lydia Pinkham's Vegetable Compound, were heavily marketed to women.[10]

Hooflander's German Bitters masked its 25 percent alcohol content behind advertising that claimed it was "entirely vegetable and free from alcoholic stimulant."[11] Similarly, the alcohol-based Great Sulphur Bitters distributed by A. R. Ordway and Company warned the public about "cheap rum drinks which are called medicine." Well-known religious and temperance leaders were used to promote these secretly laced alcoholic medicines.[12]

The first *American Pharmacopoeia,* published in 1820, contained the formulas for nine wine-based medicines. These included Wine of Ipecac, Wine of Opium, and Wine of Tobacco. In 1850, brandy and whiskey preparations were officially added to the *Pharmacopoeia.*[13] Alcohol was recommended to aid digestion, to prevent goiter, to ward off fever, and to relieve pain. Alcohol was also given to women after childbirth to help stimulate the flow of milk, and infants and children were regularly dosed with alcohol-laced medicines.[14]

By the mid-nineteenth century, the growing awareness of alcohol-related problems triggered considerable debate about the use of alcohol in medicine. Between 1872 and 1886, the American Medical Association's (AMA) House of Delegates passed four separate resolutions discouraging the use of alcoholic beverages in medicine, but physicians and pharmacists played a most curious role during the years of state and national prohibition of alcohol.

In 1917, the head of the AMA came out in favor of Prohibition, and the AMA's House of Delegates passed a resolution opposing the use of alcohol as a beverage and the use of alcohol by doctors as a therapeutic agent.[15] In spite of this resolution, the AMA was successful in getting alcohol prescribed for medical purposes listed as an exception under the Volstead Act—the act implementing national Prohibition.

In the six months following passage of the Act, 15,000 doctors and 57,000 druggists applied for licenses to prescribe and sell alcohol.[16] A 1922 AMA poll of physicians revealed that beer, ale, malt liquor, wine, whiskey, gin, and brandy were being prescribed for conditions ranging from heart attack and diabetes to snake bite.[17] By 1928, doctors were making an estimated $40 million a year writing prescriptions for whiskey.[18] Similarly, the number of pharmacies grew rapidly in the early 1920s, in great part due to the pharmacies' new role as a distributor of alcohol.[19] During America's experiment with national Prohibition, the line between medicine and intoxicant was a very thin one.

Cocaine and Other Stimulants [20]

Cocaine

Coca leaves have been chewed for their psychoactive properties for more than 4,000 years. The active ingredient in the coca shrub, *Erthroxylon coca,* was isolated by Friedrich Gaedecke in 1845 and christened "cocaine" by Albert Niemann in 1860. Cocaine was introduced into American medicine in the 1870s and was characterized in medical journals as "wholesome" and "beneficial."[21] Cocaine preparations—particularly in a solution of wine (Vin Mariani)—filled the shelves of American apothecaries and grocery stores in the 1880s, but it took a young Viennese physician to popularize the drug. His name, Sigmund Freud, is well known to this day.

In 1884, Sigmund Freud read a medical report on the use of cocaine to fight fatigue in soldiers. Intrigued, Freud ordered a supply of cocaine and began experimenting with the drug, rapidly developing an intense personal and professional fascination with cocaine. Freud shared his fascination, and his cocaine, with his fiancée, colleagues, and friends with such frenzy that his biographer would later suggest he was "rapidly becoming a public menace."[22] In 1884, the same year in which purified cocaine became available in the United States, Freud's paper "On Coca" was published in the *St. Louis Medical and Surgical Journal.* Freud set forth his view that cocaine was harmless and a great gift to humankind. He recommended cocaine as a stimulant, an aphrodisiac, an anesthetic, and a treatment for numerous medical disorders.

Cocaine was used by American physicians for many purposes but became most well known for its use as a local anesthetic in delicate surgery of the eye, nose, and throat. One of the leading pioneers of anesthesia, Dr. William Stewart Halsted, became addicted to cocaine during his early self-experiments with the drug. Cocaine-laced products were also used to treat everything from whooping cough to asthma to the common cold to masturbation.[23] One of the most troublesome uses was in the treatment of asthma and sinus conditions caused by colds and allergies. People treating these disorders used cocaine-based products repeatedly throughout the day, for prolonged periods of time. This led to increased physical tolerance and the need for ever-increasing doses.[24]

Perhaps most surprising of all, cocaine was recommended as a treatment for alcoholism and morphine addiction. As early as 1880, Kentucky physician W. H. Bentley reported that he had successfully treated alcoholism and morphine addiction using cocaine. To support this claim, he offered the case study of a woman addicted to morphine to whom he had prescribed one pound of cocaine.

> I received a note from her when she had used this. She was much encouraged and had ordered two pounds more. . . . I saw her recently when she assured me that she had no desire for morphine.[25]

Sigmund Freud made a similar claim in his 1884 paper, but he had to retract that claim when a fellow physician, whose morphine addiction Freud had treated with cocaine, became addicted to the cocaine.[26]

Cocaine became increasingly available in the 1880s as a 100-percent-pure alkaloid and in such products as Wine of Coca, Fluid Extract of Coca, Coca Cordial (cocaine and liqueur), Coca Cheroots, Coca Cigarettes, Cocaine Inhalant, Vin Mariani, Dr. Birney's Catarrh Powder, Allans Cocaine Tablets, Lloyd's Cocaine Toothache Drops, Dr. Tucker's Asthma Specific, Paine's Celery Compound, and Peruvian Wine of Coca. Cocaine-laced products came in forms designed for smoking, sniffing, and injection as well as in the form of pills, candy, gargles, and suppositories.

The advertising of some cocaine-laced products emphasized cocaine's aphrodisiac effects, its ability to restore virility, and its power as a brain stimulant for doctors, lawyers, teachers, and members of the clergy.[27] During the 1880s, fashionable women asked their doctors for cocaine injections to make themselves "lively and talkative."[28]

In the last quarter of the nineteenth century, patent medicines, tonics, and "soft drinks" were nearly indistinguishable. Cocaine was included as a central ingredient in many popular tonic drinks, including Coca Cola (which contained cocaine until 1903), Delicious Dopeless Koca Nola, Kola-Ade, Kos-Kola, Rococola, Celery Cola, Inca Cola, Wiseola, and Dope Cola.[29] Most of these products used a fluid coca extract with only one milligram of cocaine that was later replaced by caffeine.[30]

Clinical reports of cocaine toxicity and cocaine addiction began to appear in the medical literature of the 1880s and increased in the 1890s.[31] In 1885 and 1886, articles in the

New York Medical Record and the *Journal of the American Medical Association* warned of the risk of cocaine addiction by medical personnel, and reported recent case studies of cocaine-induced insanity in doctors. By 1888, warnings about cocaine were appearing in hygiene textbooks:

> Cocaine is a dangerous therapeutic toy not to be used as a sensational plaything. If it should come into as general use as other intoxicants, it will fill the asylums.[32]

By 1890, more than 400 cases of toxic cocaine reactions and more than a dozen cocaine-related deaths had been reported in the medical literature, prompting noted addiction-ologist Dr. T. D. Crothers to characterize cocainism as "a new disease of civilization."[33] In 1902, the autobiography *Eight Years in Cocaine Hell* detailed the descent of Annie Meyers from a "proper Christian woman" to a cocaine addict. It was the first confessional book about drug addiction written by an American woman.

A final note on nineteenth-century cocaine use was the observation that those addicted to cocaine often cycled into addiction to alcohol and narcotics—one of the first observations that addiction to one drug could increase vulnerability for addiction to drugs of a different class.[34]

Cocaine popularity, of course, would resurge in the twentieth century, most dramatically in the 1980s. Cocaine use re-emerged at a time the drug was viewed as non-addicting and relatively harmless.[35] Ironically and tragically, reports on cocaine-related toxicity, deaths, and addiction in the 1980s bear striking similarity to those reported in the addictions literature of the 1880s.

Amphetamine and Psychostimulants

Other stimulants that came to be used in medicine shared a similar fate as cocaine.[36] Amphetamine was synthesized in 1887 and first used medically to treat asthma in 1912. Gordon Alles's research in the 1920s on the effects of amphetamine and the release of the first commercial amphetamine—the Benzedrine inhaler—in 1932 set the stage for widespread medical use. Amphetamines were first used to treat depression, obesity, narcolepsy (a disorder that produces sudden, brief, uncontrollable sleep during the day), congestion (of asthma, colds, and hay fever), epilepsy, schizophrenia, enuresis (bed wetting), migraine headaches, and alcoholism.

In 1937, Charles Bradley reported that amphetamines improved the learning and overall behavior of hyperactive children. Benzedrine was followed by the introduction of other amphetamines (such as Dexedrine) and psychostimulants (such as Ritalin and Cylert) that became widely used. The use of Ritalin in the treatment of hyperactivity became so widespread among school children in the United States during the late twentieth century that some observers began to refer to the "three Rs" as "reading, writing, and Ritalin."

The first report of amphetamine misuse occurred in 1936 when students used in experiments on the drug conducted at the University of Minnesota began seeking out the drug on their own. Knowledge of amphetamine's effects became widely known in the American culture of the 1940s, as evidenced by the popularity of the song "Who Put the Benzedrine in Mrs. Murphy's Ovaltine."[37] Although most of the people receiving medical prescriptions for amphetamines were women and children, amphetamines (many acquired from a growing black market) also became popular among athletes, business executives, truck drivers, and students during the 1940s. Reports of amphetamine overdoses prompted the removal of the Benzedrine inhaler from the market in 1949.

As the 1960s approached, amphetamines and related psychostimulants were frequently prescribed for weight control, with some "fat doctors" distributing massive quantities of these drugs upon request. Such doctors were responsible for addicting large numbers of women to amphetamines, and they were the initial source of amphetamines diverted to the illicit drug culture in the 1960s.[38] As amphetamines were diverted to and synthesized within a growing illicit drug culture of the late 1960s, there was particular concern about the practice of injecting methamphetamine (Methedrine or Desoxyn)—a practice that cycled into narcotic and sedative addiction by the mid-1970s.

Marijuana

Recent debate over the use of marijuana (cannabis) in American medicine obscures the long history of such use. Marijuana entered American medicine in the 1840s and 1850s and was first listed in the official *Pharmacopoeia* in 1873.[39] Most often available as a tincture (cannabis suspended in alcohol), the drug was prescribed for a wide variety of medical conditions, including loss of appetite, coughing, insomnia, seizures, venereal infections, tetanus, anxiety, menstrual problems, depression, migraine headaches, and alcohol and narcotic withdrawal.[40]

While many doctors praised the drug's potential in medicine, its detractors focused on the variability and unpredictability of potency—a problem that led to no effects or unpleasant side effects. The use of cannabis in medicine declined due to the introduction of alternative drugs, but cannabis-based products did not disappear. At the time of the anti-marijuana campaign of the 1930s and the drug's prohibition in 1937, it was still available in more than twenty-five pharmaceutical preparations, including such over-the-counter products as Piso's Cure, One Day Cough Cure, and Neurosine.[41]

Cannabis, mostly in the form of hashish, began to be used in America for its intoxicating properties in the second half of the nineteenth century. The first American account of cannabis use was Bayard Taylor's reports on hashish in his 1854 and 1855 books, *A Journey to Central Africa* and *The Lands of the Saracen*.[42] Fitz Hugh Ludlow, a minister's son, was so struck by Taylor's descriptions that he began his own experiments with a cannabis extract procured from a local apothecary. Ludlow's experiences with marijuana were published in an 1857 article in *Putnam's Magazine* and later expanded into the book *The Hasheesh Eater*.[43] It was in Ludlow's writings that most Americans of this period first became aware of the euphorigenic properties of marijuana.

Reports of American Hashish Clubs frequented by writers and artists first appeared in the popular press of the late 1850s. By 1876, "hashish house" exposés began to appear in magazines like the *Illustrated Police Gazette* under such titles as "Secret Dissipation of New York Belles: Interior of a Hashish Hell on Fifth Avenue."[44] There are only a few such reports of cannabis use in the last half of the nineteenth century, suggesting that experimentation with the drug was not widespread. The Harrison Narcotics Tax Act of 1914, which controlled opiates and cocaine, did not include marijuana, in spite of testimony by addiction experts like Dr. Alexander Lambert that marijuana was habit-forming. The drug was excluded because it had little visibility in the culture at that time and because of physicians' lobbying that the drug should remain available as a medicine.

The practice of smoking marijuana came to the United States with Mexican migrant workers in the 1920s[45] and slowly seeped into the bohemian fringes of American culture.[46] Mid-twentieth-century Americans learned of the drug through the occasional report of a jazz musician's arrest or through musical references to marijuana, such as "That Old Reefer Man," "Sweet Marijuana," "Sweet Marihuana Brown," and "Viper's Drag."[47]

Marijuana emerged in the 1960s and 1970s as a celebrated drug within the American youth culture, peaked in the late 1970s, declined through the early 1980s, and then rose again in the 1990s. Through these peaks and valleys of use, the debate over the role of marijuana in medicine has continued. In 1985, the Food and Drug Administration (FDA) gave approval to Unimed, Inc., a New Jersey–based research company, to produce Marinol, a THC derivative used in the treatment of nausea often experienced by patients receiving chemotherapy. The use of marijuana in medicine continues to be hotly debated, with several states having passed laws allowing its use to treat such conditions as glaucoma, to stimulate appetite, and to treat the side effects of chemotherapy.

Sedatives and Barbiturates

Bromides and Chloral

There is a long history of the use of sedatives and barbiturates in American medicine. The first such drugs were the bromide salts, whose ability to produce sedation brought them growing popularity during the 1870s.[48] It wasn't long, however, before physicians discovered that bromides brought the risk of accidental poisoning (overdose) and addiction. The bromides were followed by chloral hydrate, best known to the general public as the "Mickey Finn" or the "knock-out drops" of detective stories. It came into widespread use following discovery of its sedating properties in 1869.[49]

An ancestor of the barbiturates (and eventually replaced by them), chloral was known as an excellent "soporific" (sleep-inducing) drug and was also used in the treatment of nervous and mental disorders.[50] The addiction potential of chloral hydrate was first reported by Dr. B. W. Richardson of London in 1871, and reports of chloral addiction, particularly among women, became common in the 1880s.[51] Chloral addiction in women continued to be reflected in early twentieth-century literature, as in Edith Wharton's *The House of Mirth*.

Paraldehyde

Paraldehyde, a non-barbiturate sedative liquid with a strong odor and bitter taste, was discovered in 1829 and later (in 1881) introduced into medicine. It was used in the treatment of alcoholic withdrawal until it was replaced by barbiturates, and then by benzodiazepines. Although a few reports of paraldehyde use for intoxication did surface over the years, particularly reports of its use by alcoholics, its unpleasant smell and taste diminished its attractiveness as an intoxicant.

Barbiturates

Barbituric acid was first used in medicine in 1882, but it was not used as a sedative until barbitone was released commercially in 1903 under the trade name Veronal. A second barbiturate, phenobarbital, was introduced in 1912 under the trade name Luminal. Two American chemists, Shonle and Moment, pioneered the procedures that made possible the inexpensive manufacture of a large number of barbiturate derivatives.[52] More than a thousand barbiturate compounds were eventually developed, about fifty of which became commercial medicines used to help people sleep or calm themselves during the daytime.

Problems of drug dependence resulting from barbiturate use developed slowly and invisibly over decades. Charles B. Towns, who operated an addiction treatment hospital in New York City, declared in 1912 that these new "hypnotics" were habit-forming and should be legally controlled.[53] In 1937, the American Medical Association issued a report entitled "Evils from Promiscuous Use of Barbituric Acid and Derivative Drugs." The report voiced concern about the rising number of accidental deaths related to barbiturate use and the rising number of barbiturate-related suicides.[54]

In 1940, one forth of American hospital admissions for poisoning were due to acute barbiturate intoxication. In the early 1950s, American medical literature recognized the addictive properties of barbiturates, identified their withdrawal syndrome and medical complications, and outlined procedures for medical detoxification. Shorter-acting barbiturates sold under such trade names as Amytal, Nembutal, Seconal, and Tuinal broke into cultural visibility in the 1960s with reports of their widespread misuse.

Thalidomide

Among the many new sedatives and tranquilizers that came on the market in the 1950s was a sedative sold in Europe under the name Contergan. Its reputation as a sleep aid, its lack of side effects, and its low price made it popular. The drug was widely sold in many countries, and in 1960, an application was filed with the federal FDA to sell the drug in the United States under the name thalidomide. All of the supporting documentation spoke glowingly of the drug's safety and the benefits of its use,[55] but medical resistance held up the drug's approval in the United States.

It was subsequently discovered that Contergan/thalidomide

produced more than 5,000 cases of severe physical deformity in babies born to the mostly European women who had used it. Thalidomide's potentially devastating effects were very difficult to identify because those effects occurred only if the mother had used the drug during a brief, specific point in the pregnancy. The fact that pregnant women who took thalidomide at other times delivered normal children helped mask thalidomide's more malignant effects.[56]

Quaalude

Growing concern about the abuse potential of barbiturates led to the search for non-addicting sedatives. New drugs such as ethchlovynol (Placidyl) and glutethimide (Doriden) vied for this lucrative niche in American medicine. One of the most promising of the non-barbiturate sedatives was methaqualone. Synthesized in 1951, methaqualone was introduced into American medicine in the mid-1960s under such trade names as Quaalude, Sopor, and Mecquin. Its designation as a Schedule V drug indicated a low potential for abuse and allowed unlimited refills. Marketed as a non-addicting substitute for barbiturates, Quaalude quickly became one of the top selling sedatives in the country. By 1968, medical reports of physical dependence, toxicity, and overdose deaths produced by methaqualone appeared and autobiographical accounts of Quaalude addiction were published.[57]

Methaqualone manufactured in illicit laboratories entered the illicit drug market in the early 1970s. The growing evidence of its misuse prompted federal authorities in 1973 to move methaqualone from Schedule V to Schedule II—indicating its high addiction potential. The excessive prescribing of methaqualone through so-called stress clinics in Florida led the state legislature to move the drug to Schedule I, banning its legal use in medicine within the state.

The excessive use of stimulants and sedatives often produced concurrent cycles of stimulants during the day and sedatives at night. The propensity for chemically induced daily cycles of sedation and stimulation became a focus of medical concern and a subject of the popular 1960s book and movie *Valley of the Dolls*.

Nitrous Oxide, Chloroform, and Ether

Nitrous oxide was introduced into dentistry and surgery by Dr. Horace Wells in 1844. Wells subsequently became addicted to chloroform and committed suicide in 1849 after an episode of intoxication during which he was arrested for throwing acid on prostitutes.[58] Occasional reports of nitrous oxide use for intoxication have continued to appear in the intervening years, including sensational reports of rich women treating their party guests with samples of nitrous oxide.[59]

Chloroform was separately discovered in 1831 by Samuel Guthrie in America and Justus von Liebig in Germany,[60] and it went on to play a significant role as a surgical anesthetic. Inhaling chloroform as an intoxicant became a fad in the 1850s. Confessional accounts of its misuse appeared in medical journals of the 1880s. These accounts described early chloroform intoxication as "love at first site" and a "heaven of chaste pleasures" and ended with tales of the user's self-deception and gradual slide into "chloroformomania."[61] Dr. T. D. Crothers noted that women were more vulnerable to chloroform addiction than men.[62]

Ether was first synthesized in 1541 and rediscovered by the German physician Friedrich Hoffmann in 1730.[63] Hoffmann christened his liquid form of ether "anodyne" and recommended it for pain. Ether was first introduced for surgical anesthesia in 1846 by William Morton who discovered its properties while observing medical students participating in "ether frolics."[64] The first medical report on ether addiction appeared in an 1847 *Lancet* article describing a gentleman whose ether use progressed so far beyond his control that he needed "permanent restraint."[65] The use of ether as an intoxicant became particularly popular in Ireland in the 1840s, an epidemic blamed on a local physician who liberally prescribed ether mixed in water.[66]

The Arsenic Eaters

Perhaps one of the strangest patterns of drug use in the late nineteenth and early twentieth centuries was that of arsenic eating. It seems strange that people could become addicted to eating what is today known as a poison, but arsenic was used in medicine, both as a tonic and as a remedy for disorders such as psoriasis. People began taking arsenic in ever-increasing quantities to gain everything from improved appearance and increased strength to sexual excitability. Problems arose when tolerance reached toxic levels or when users who suddenly stopped taking arsenic went into life-threatening withdrawal. Studies of habitual arsenic users noted that this pattern was common in the southern United States, where arsenic eaters were called "Dippers."[67]

Tranquilizers

A psychopharmacological revolution unfolded in the 1950s. The introduction of chlorpromazine in 1954 as the first "major tranquilizer" radically changed the treatment of schizophrenia and other serious mental illness. This change sparked interest in the synthesis of new mind-altering drugs ("minor tranquilizers") that could treat milder forms of mental distress, particularly anxiety. The story of a class of drugs known as benzodiazepines begins with the drug meprobamate, which was synthesized in England in 1950. Meprobamate was introduced into American medicine in 1955 under the trade names Miltown and Equanil. These were the first effective and widely available antianxiety agents.

The rapid recognition of their dependence potential sparked the search for alternatives. More than 3,000 benzodiazepine compounds were subsequently created, with about twenty-five used clinically in medicine. The breakthrough came with the 1960 discovery of Librium. It rose in popularity only to be eclipsed by Valium in 1963. Subsequent generations of benzodiazepine research produced new anti-anxiety agents such as Ativan and Xanax.[68] As a group, these drugs have been called anxiolytics, antineurotic agents, or antianxiety agents.[69]

The use of benzodiazepine drugs increased because of their benign reputation. However, there were objections to the practice of designating these drugs as "minor tranquilizers." Some psychiatrists thought the term belittled and undermined the seriousness of the disorders these drugs were used to treat. Addiction specialists criticized such designation on the grounds that it contributed to the illusion that these substances were not powerful and potentially addictive. Studies in the 1960s confirmed the potential for physical dependence on benzodiazepines and case reports of such dependence had been reported for the past thirty years.[70] One of the most vivid portrayals of Valium addiction is contained in Barbara Gordon's 1979 book, *I'm Dancing As Fast As I Can*.

LSD, PCP, and Ecstasy (MDMA)

There are numerous early reports of the use of hallucinogens within Native American spiritual and healing rituals. There are also a few early twentieth-century reports of mescaline experimentation by S. Weir Mitchell, a prominent American psychiatrist and writer, and Havelock Ellis, an English psychologist.[71] However, the story of the use of hallucinogens in Western medicine begins primarily with the discovery of LSD.

LSD

The story of LSD begins with ergot, a parasitic fungus that grows on rye and other grains. Periodic outbreaks of ergot poisoning, accompanied by hallucinations and extreme disorientation, had been reported since the fourteenth century. These outbreaks usually followed the consumption of ergot-contaminated bread. Beginning in the sixteenth century, ergot compounds were used in small doses to relieve pain, stop bleeding, and start uterine contractions. In the early 1930s, the common ingredient of the ergot alkaloids was identified as lysergic acid.[72]

In 1938, two chemists at Sandoz Laboratories in Basel, Switzerland, Dr. Albert Hofmann and Dr. Arthur Stoll, created a series of ergot compounds in an effort to synthesize a pain remedy for migraine headaches. Working with lysergic acid isolated from the ergot, Hofmann added a diethylamine molecule. The twenty-fifth compound in the series was d-lysergic acid diethylamide tartrate, or "LSD 25." Research on LSD 25 and its chemical cousins ceased in 1938 as there appeared to be no use for the substances. Five years later, Hofmann again synthesized LSD 25 and accidentally ingested a tiny amount of the drug. Hofmann's error led not only to the discovery of a new drug but also to discovery of a totally new type of drug, whose chemical structure and profound psychoactive effects from miniscule doses had never before been seen.

In 1947, the psychiatrist Dr. Werner Stoll (Dr. Arthur

Stoll's son) obtained a supply of LSD from Sandoz Laboratories and began the first controlled human experiments with the drug.[73] In 1949, LSD was delivered to more than ninety researchers wishing to experiment with the drug in the treatment of psychiatric illness and alcoholism. Between 1949 and the mid-1960s, many researchers and psychotherapists used LSD in the treatment of alcoholism, childhood autism, impotence and frigidity, neuroses, character disorders, anticipatory grief (of those facing death), and pathological mourning.

With careful patient selection and adequate preparation and supervision, they found they could minimize the risks of adverse reactions.[74] Popular accounts, such as a 1959 *Look* magazine article attributing Cary Grant's newfound happiness to LSD psychotherapy, spurred great interest in the drug. While early anecdotal reports fired optimism about the future of this new drug in the field of psychiatry, later controlled studies showed less dramatic results. The growing controversy related to LSD's widespread misuse in the 1960s and subsequent documentation of its adverse effects led to the legal prohibition of LSD and most other known hallucinogens.

PCP

Another hallucinogen that started out in medicine but became best known for its adverse effects in the illicit drug culture was phencyclidine, widely known as PCP. PCP was developed in the early 1950s and introduced into medicine in 1959 under the trade name Sernyl. The drug seemed to have great promise as a surgical anesthetic. It produced a rapid loss of consciousness and lessened post-surgical pain. The problem was that about 15 percent of patients receiving the drug awoke from anesthesia in a state of profound disorientation resembling schizophrenia. Due to these toxic reactions, the drug's use with humans was banned, and further legal availability was restricted to its use as an immobilizer of upper primates in veterinary medicine. PCP arrived in the illicit drug culture in the late 1960s, and its use increased into the late 1970s at which time its popularity waned amidst reports of PCP-induced psychoses.[75]

Ecstasy (MDMA)

A drug possessing both stimulant and hallucinogenic properties that transitioned from medical use to illicit use was the substance known today as Ecstasy. MDMA was first developed as a potential diet aid in 1914 in Germany but it was discontinued due to adverse side effects. It first appeared in the illicit drug culture in 1970 but never gained the popularity of LSD. During the early 1980s, the drug was used as an adjunct in psychotherapy in a manner similar to earlier work with LSD. As a result of reports of positive experiences with the drug in this setting, interest in the drug increased, which resulted in the drug's re-emergence in the illicit drug market. In 1985, the Drug Enforcement Administration (DEA) used its emergency powers to place Ecstasy in Schedule I, designating a high potential for abuse and high penalties for its possession or sale.

The Story of "Poppers"

Amyl nitrate is a yellowish, fruity-smelling liquid that rapidly decomposes through evaporation. It was discovered by Ascanio Sobrero in 1847 and introduced into medicine in 1867 to treat angina pectoris—a treatment that capitalized on the drug's ability to dilate coronary arteries and oxygenate heart muscle.

Marketed under such brand names as Vaporole and Aspirole, amyl nitrate came in small glass pearls surrounded by absorbent fibers that were broken open and the vapors inhaled. The use of amyl nitrate and butyl nitrate in medicine decreased as more preferred vasodilators such as nitroglycerin became available.

The first reports of the inhalation of amyl nitrate for intoxication dates to the 1930s but increased rapidly in the late 1970s. As the demand increased for "poppers" (a name derived from the sound made when they are broken), new amyl nitrate products came onto the market under such trade names as Rush, Locker Room, Aroma of Men, Kick, and Jac Aroma.

Narcotics

Opium

Opium came to America early and in many forms. There was raw prepared opium. There was granulated opium, prepared in standard medical doses and taken by mouth, usually to treat diarrhea. There was powdered opium, the fine granules of which could be sprinkled into an open wound to relieve pain. There was tincture of opium: opium suspended in alcohol. Three of the earliest and most popular opium products were Laudanum, Paregoric, and Dover's Powder.[76]

Laudanum, originally in the form of an opium pill and later in a liquid combination of opium and alcohol, was developed by Paracelsus, a Swiss chemist, in the sixteenth century. In colonial America, the term *laudanum* was used for a number of preparations that combined opium with ingredients such as wine, henbane, bone of the heart of a stag, cinnamon, frog's sperm, and orange or lemon juice. The alcoholic preparation of opium that people drank was the most popular[77] and was regularly used by such prominent Americans as Benjamin Franklin.[78]

Paregoric—a mixture of opium, alcohol, camphor, benzoic acid, and anise oil—appeared in the early eighteenth century and was the most common product recommended for diarrhea.

Paregoric was also one of the most frequently used medicines for children.

Dover's Powder was an opium-based preparation developed by Dr. Thomas Dover of England for the treatment of gout. It contained a concoction of opium, licorice, ipecac, and other assorted ingredients. Dover's Powder was used as a painkiller, usually taken internally or applied to the skin.

There are only a few early reports of opium addiction from the colonial period. Jan Huyghen van Linschoten, describing his own opium use on a voyage to the West Indies during the colonial period, noted:

> He that useth to eate it, must eate it daylie, otherwise he dieth and consumeth himself. . . . He that hath never eaten it, and will venture at first to eate as much as those that daylie use it, it will surely kill him.[79]

During the early 1800s, new opium-based products were popular in America, including "black-drop" (also known as Lancaster or Quaker's Black-drop) and Dr. Barton's "brown mixture," a combination of opium and licorice.

The 1832 medical dissertation of Dr. William Smith observed that opium "is in every day's use, and particularly among the better circles of society, and by the softer sex,"[80] but there are few references to opiate addiction in the medical and popular literature before 1860. Five factors set the stage for the dramatic rise in opiate addiction in the closing decades of the nineteenth century: 1) epidemic diseases, 2) the introduction of morphine, 3) the invention of the hypodermic syringe, 4) the Civil War, and 5) an aggressive patent medicine industry.[81]

The cholera epidemics of 1832–1833, 1848, and 1854, and

the sustained spread of dysentery between 1847 and 1851 were all commonly treated with opiates.[82] As late as 1913, Dr. George Pettey was reporting that opium and morphine were used to treat chronic rheumatism, migraine headaches, liver and kidney disease, asthma, chronic dysentery, hookworm, pellagra, tuberculosis, cancer, and alcoholism; these uses were the primary source of the spread of narcotic addiction.[83]

Morphine

In 1805, the German chemist Friedrich Sertürner isolated morphine from opium. Sertürner christened his new drug after Morpheus, the Greek god of sleep.[84] Morphine was introduced into American medicine in 1825 and was in widespread use by physicians in the 1830s.[85] This technical breakthrough delivered an opiate product of unprecedented potency that became a universal antidote for pain. By the 1850s, morphine-based products filled the shelves of America's drugstores where citizens could buy them over-the-counter without a prescription. Morphine was used in place of opium out of the widespread belief that it lacked opium's addictive properties.[86]

As early as 1656–1657, Christopher Wren, a professor of astronomy at Gresham College in London, experimented with the process of injecting drugs directly into the veins of animals and human beings, but it was left to Irish surgeon Francis Rynd (1844) and Scottish physician Alexander Wood (1853) to develop a workable method and instrument for the hypodermic injection of medicines.

The hypodermic syringe was introduced into the United States just before the Civil War.[87] Unlike earlier methods, the syringe provided an extremely efficient way of administering opiates—a method so efficient that its promoters claimed it could reduce the risks of addiction because injection could alleviate pain with smaller quantities of morphine than other methods. In fact, Wood did not believe that morphine would be addictive if it were injected. Tragically, his wife was one of the first people to die from an overdose of morphine administered by hypodermic syringe.

One of the first articles signaling alarm about addiction from injection of morphine was a T. C. Albutt report in the *Lancet* in 1864. Such reports became common in the 1870s when hypodermic drug use gained wide popularity. In 1879, in his text, *The Hypodermic Method,* Dr. Robert Bartholow warned of the following dire consequence of this new invention:

> The introduction of the hypodermic has placed in the hands of man a means of intoxication more seductive than any which has heretofore contributed to his craving for narcotic stimulation. So common now are the instances of habitual use, and so enslaving is the habit when indulged in by this mode, that a lover of mankind must regard the future with no little apprehension.[88]

Controversy surrounds the role of the Civil War in the rise of narcotic addiction in the United States. The traditionalist view is that the Civil War played a major role in the spread of narcotic addiction, which became known as the "soldier's disease." According to this view, narcotic addiction was spawned by thousands of soldiers who became addicted to the injected morphine used to treat their wounds.[89] There are some memoirs of addicted Civil War veterans *(Opium Eating: An Autobiographical Sketch; Doctor Judas)* that support this view. An opposing view comes from modern historians who conclude that the Civil War did contribute to the rise of addiction, but that much of that addiction occurred not during but after the war—when morphine and the hypodermic syringe became more widely available.[90]

What no historian argues is the role the patent medicine industry played in the spread of narcotic addiction in the late nineteenth century. Although opium was available in crude form during the eighteenth century, it was not until the nineteenth century that a patent medicine industry arose, with opiate-filled elixirs and nostrums as the centerpiece of its offerings. The most popular opium-laced patent medicines included Paregoric Elixir (camphorated tincture of opium), Perkin's Diarrhea Mixture, McMunn's Elixir of Opium, and Ayer's Cherry Pectoral.

Opiate-based medicines were available from doctors, drugstores (without a prescription), grocery stores, mail-order houses, and traveling peddlers who went from town to town selling their chemical wares. In his autobiographical account of addiction, William Cobbe wrote about buying opiates in drugstores "which sell the poison as indifferently as they sell toilet soap."[91]

Dr. David Musto has investigated the role of the physician in the spread of opiate addiction in the nineteenth century. He concludes that physicians played an *inadvertent* role by prescribing a new product like heroin (which was not yet known to be addictive), a *negligent* role by prescribing narcotics in fear the patient would simply seek another doctor if refused, or an *intentional* role in cases where physicians consciously addicted alcoholics to morphine on the grounds that morphine was less harmful than alcohol.[92]

The best evidence of the growth in American opiate use can be found in the annual figures for importation of opium, figures kept quite carefully for tax purposes. The volume of crude opium and smoking opium imported into the United States rose from 450,925 pounds during the 1840s to more than 6 million pounds during the 1890s. Annual per capita opium consumption rose from 12 grains in 1840 to 52 grains in 1890.[93]

In their classic work, *The Opium Problem,* Charles Terry and Mildred Pellens concluded that most opiate addicts in the second half of the nineteenth century and the early twentieth century were white, middle-aged, educated, affluent women living in the rural South. The stories of these culturally invisible addicted women were occasionally revealed through such literary works as Harper Lee's *To Kill a Mockingbird* and Eugene O'Neill's *Long Day's Journey into Night.* The high rate of narcotic addiction in women was also evident in rising medical reports of neonatal narcotic addiction in the 1880s and 1890s.[94]

The patent medicine industry targeted children as well as women with its products. Some opium- and cocaine-laced patent medicines were promoted specifically for use with babies. Dr. J. C. Fahey's Pepsin Anodyne claimed to "pacify the most fretful child." Promising that the product contained "no laudanum or injurious article," the Fahey preparation contained both chloral hydrate and morphine.[95]

Opiate-laced preparations in products like Mrs. Winslow's Soothing Syrup, Godfrey's Cordial, Children's Comfort, Mother Bailey's Quieting Syrup, Steedman's Teething Powders, Paregoric Elixir, and Hooper's Anodyne ("The Infant's Friend") were so popular for calming infants and children that warnings began to appear about their potentially deadly effects.[96]

Dr. J. B. Mattison, America's foremost nineteenth-century authority on narcotic addiction, regularly voiced his conviction that morphinism in babies and children was far more widespread than people believed, and that this condition played a hidden role in America's infant mortality rate.[97]

Nineteenth century medical literature also portrayed addiction as an occupational vulnerability of nurses, doctors, and doctors' spouses. In an 1883 article on opium addiction among physicians, Mattison blamed this vulnerability on their access to the drug, their intimate knowledge of the hypodermic, and the weary days and sleepless nights that typified the life of the physician.[98] In 1899, Dr. T. D. Crothers estimated that 10 percent of American physicians were addicted to narcotic drugs.[99]

Heroin

Diacetylmorphine was originally synthesized by the London chemist C. R. Alder Wright in 1874, but it did not enter medical use until 1898. Heroin was introduced as a non-addictive alternative to morphine and codeine and advertised and displayed in drugstores next to Aspirin (introduced in 1899). Heroin was initially used to treat coughs, asthma, bronchitis, emphysema, and tuberculosis, but subsequently gained popularity with a new breed of urban addict. Addicts like Leroy Street bought heroin over the counter without a prescription before the drug was banned. In his autobiography, *I Was a Drug Addict,* Street described how drugstores would give their regular addicts a present each Christmas: a shiny new hypodermic syringe wrapped in a red ribbon, with a Christmas card attached.[100]

Opium and morphine were associated with the relief of pain, but heroin came to be associated with the search for pleasure. Most nineteenth-century opiate addicts traced the beginning of their addiction to doctors' prescriptions or to self-medication of ailments with opiate-laced patent medicines, but by 1914, only 20 of 1,000 narcotic addicts treated at the City Prison in Manhattan cited physician-prescribed opiates as the original source of their addiction.[101]

Concern about the growing problem of narcotic addiction and the changing profile of the narcotic addict stirred social reformers. The result was a demand for stricter controls on narcotic drugs. The controls took several forms: passage of state prescription laws (or laws requiring that pharmacists sell drugs only for legitimate purposes); passage of the federal Pure Food and Drug Act of 1906, which required that products containing alcohol, opium, and cocaine be so labeled; and passage of federal legislation (the 1914 Harrison Narcotics Tax Act) that marked the beginning of the criminalization of addiction in America.

As the twentieth century progressed, new synthetic narcotics were introduced into medicine—drugs like Dilaudid, Metapon, Dionin, Pantopon, Percodan, Dromoran, Leritine, Prinadol, and Demerol. Like their predecessors, many of these drugs were believed to be non-addicting at the time they were introduced into medical practice but later proved to have high addiction liability.

When narcotic addicts lost their ability to maintain access to narcotics, either as a result of personal circumstances or disruptions in local illicit drug markets, there were frantic attempts to find a substitute that could stave off narcotic withdrawal. These experiments, often involving efforts to entice various drugs from physicians, generated their own new drug trends.

T's and Blues

The mid-1970s was a strange time for heroin addicts on the streets of Chicago. The traditional trafficking channels that had placed a low-grade but consistently available Asian heroin on the streets of Chicago were breaking up and giving way to new channels that were delivering Mexican brown heroin. During this transition, there were days when heroin was difficult to find. Sick addicts began experimenting with almost any drug or drug combination that would medicate their discomfort. Such experimentation led to the discovery of a heroin substitute that became pervasive among Chicago heroin users and then spread to other cities with large addict populations. The heroin substitute, known on the streets as "T's and Blues," was a combination of pentazocine (a synthetic painkiller marketed under the trade name Talwin) and Pyribenzamine, a common antihistamine found in many over-the-counter medicines.

The two drugs were crushed and mixed together in solution, "cooked," and injected intravenously like heroin. Addicts capitalized on the synergistic interaction between the two drugs—an effect not predictable from either drug's known effects. "T's and Blues" continued as a phenomenon until Talwin was brought under greater legal control, via placement in Schedule II, and the accessibility of heroin returned.[102]

China White and MPTP
"Designer drugs"—a term coined by pharmacologist Gary Henderson—represent efforts by chemists to alter the molecular structure of a psychoactive drug to change the drug identity while maintaining or intensifying the original drug's psychoactive properties. Designer drugs are *analogues,* chemical cousins of their originals, and may have effects and risks quite different than the original substance. Motivations to create such products include their legal status. Before 1986, such chemical cousins were not illegal to possess or sell and were often undetectable through routine urine testing.

The modern story of designer drugs begins in 1976 with a bright, twenty-three-year-old college student from Bethesda, Maryland, who was addicted to meperidine (Demerol). Desiring to continue using Demerol but fearing legal apprehension, he prepared MPPP, a chemical cousin of Demerol that was not legally controlled. He continued to synthesize and use MPPP for six months without incident. In the summer of 1976, he prepared a new batch of the drug, but a mistake in the synthesis procedure produced not MPPP, but a highly potent neurotoxin: MPTP. Following ingestion of MPTP, the young college student suffered partial paralysis, muscle spasms and tremors, slowness of movement, a mask-like face, and a loss of speech. He had, in short, developed what appeared to be the classic symptoms of Parkinson's disease that did not fully remit over time. His story might have been easily lost to history if it were not for future developments.[103]

In 1979, two California men were found dead with fresh needle tracks and drug injection paraphernalia and white powder close to their bodies. The DEA's Washington lab identified the powder as a designer narcotic. Deaths from "synthetic heroin" continued to be reported through 1980 and 1981. Then in the summer of 1982, a completely new chapter of this story unfolded in southern California. Following the Fourth of July weekend, neurologist J. William Langston treated a forty-year-old patient brought to Santa Clara Valley Medical Center. The patient had symptoms precisely like those described above in our young college student, and a week later, the girlfriend of Langston's patient experienced the same parkinsonian symptoms. Within three weeks, Langston had treated seven drug users with what appeared to be advanced Parkinson's disease.

Analysis of the drugs Langston's patients had used confirmed the presence of MPTP—obtained in heroin sold under the name "China White."[104] Langston's analysis of this phenomenon included a dire warning: in some users, the MPTP may have only partially damaged the substantia nigra, which would not reveal active symptoms immediately but could reveal those symptoms later through the aging process. In short, some users could already have set a course that would unfold the onset of Parkinson's disease in the next five to ten years.[105]

Fentanyl Analogues

Other designer narcotics marked the introduction of fentanyl analogues into the illicit drug supply. Fentanyl is a synthetic narcotic introduced into American medicine under the brand name Sublimaze in 1972. It is widely used in surgery to produce short-term anesthesia. Its availability and potency have been linked to the dramatic rise in addiction among anesthesiologists and nurse anesthetists in the United States.

While there was early evidence of fentanyl addiction among medical personnel, fentanyl was not expected to be a candidate for illicit diversion because of its short duration of effect. This problem was solved in 1979 when a "phantom chemist" created two fentanyl analogues that were longer acting. These analogues—alpha-methyl fentanyl and 3-methyl fentanyl—approached the duration of effect of heroin.[106] The potency of the more than 200 known fentanyl analogues is quite remarkable. The two most common analogues named above are, respectively, 200 and 1,000 times more potent than morphine.

Fentanyl analogues appeared within the illicit drug culture as early as December 1979, and by 1981, treatment centers were encountering self-proclaimed heroin addicts entering treatment whose urine samples did not test positive for opiates. It was later confirmed that these clients had been using "China

White" or other products sold as "synthetic heroin." Use of designer opiates increased during the mid-1980s. Melanie Kirsch reported in 1986 that 10 percent of clients in northern California methadone clinics tested positive for fentanyl derivatives when special tests for fentanyl were administered for all incoming clients. The number of cases of MPTP-induced Parkinson's disease also rose.[107]

By 1985, the Centers for Disease Control and Prevention (CDC) had identified 400 MPTP-exposed individuals. These individuals presented with symptoms such as lost or impaired speech, impaired mobility (slow, stooped gait), stiffness, and tremors. The CDC also reported more than 100 deaths related to designer opiates.[108] Some of the fentanyl overdose deaths were caused by synergistic interaction between fentanyl analogues and other drugs, particularly cocaine and alcohol. Dr. Richard Restak, commenting on the historical significance of designer drugs, notes the thin line between benefit and injury and that the most minute modification in a drug's structure can "unleash powerful unintended forces."[109]

Lessons of History

There are many lessons that can be drawn from the brief history we have reviewed. Here are some of the most significant.[110]

There is an unrelenting quality in the relationship between human beings and psychoactive drugs. Humans always have and probably always will use psychoactive drugs to alter their consciousness; alleviate physical, emotional, and spiritual distress; and express their identification with particular social groups. Psychoactive drugs have brought great blessings to human beings, but those gifts can bring harmful effects that must be actively managed by individuals, communities, and countries.

A psychoactive drug can lie dormant within a culture and within the practice of medicine for a long time before it emerges as a drug linked to serious substance-use problems and addiction. The implication of this principle is that future drugs that will generate the attention that OxyContin has recently received are already here and we do not yet recognize them. The globalization of drug tastes, which will bring intoxicants from other cultures into American medicine and the illicit drug culture, will dramatically expand the American psychoactive drug menu.

Several strategies have proved effective in containing emerging drug epidemics. Prescription laws, product labeling laws, and improved physician training in the late nineteenth and early twentieth centuries dramatically reduced the rate of narcotic addiction resulting from medical treatment. Clearly designating drugs with a high potential for abuse, educating physicians about the risk of drug dependence, monitoring physician prescribing practices, and attempting to prevent the illicit manufacture and distribution of psychoactive drugs used in medicine have also proved effective in containing surges in problems related to amphetamine, barbiturate, and non-barbiturate sedative dependence. Drug control strategies are not a complete failure as is sometimes portrayed, but such successes can be time-limited.

Drugs with great potential for misuse go through cycles of popularity and hibernation, only to resurface later, usually in a more virulent pattern. These cyclical trends are clearly evident in the history of stimulant and narcotic addiction in the United States. Periods of intense consumption of short-acting stimulants are often followed by a brief transition to long-acting stimulants and then by increased consumption of alcohol, sedatives, and narcotics. The rampant cocaine and methamphetamine use of the 1980s and 1990s set the stage for the increased opiate use (both heroin and prescription narcotics) that followed it. Those communities that are now plagued with problems related to methamphetamine use but have never witnessed problems of narcotic addiction should be aware of their increasing vulnerability for the latter.

When drugs first emerge or re-emerge, some of the first casualties related to the drug can be found among those closest to the drug's emergence and popularization, for example, the drug's discoverers, physicians, and pharmacists. These professionals and their inner circle of family, friends, and colleagues have often been victimized by miscalculations of the risk inherent within the new or modified substance or the new methods through which it is ingested.

Any change in potency, form, or method of administration of a drug may dramatically alter its addiction potential. The isolation of morphine, the introduction of new forms of cocaine, and the introduction of the hypodermic syringe all illustrate this principle. A drug may be relatively safe at one dose but have a high potential for misuse at another, may have a low potential for misuse when consumed orally but a high potential for misuse when ingested intranasally or by injection. In short, slight changes in the character of an existing drug and how the drug is administered could force a radical rethinking of the nature and dangers associated with the drug.

Some drugs enter the culture as a Trojan horse, masking their dangers to a minority of citizens in the benefits they bring to the majority. The fact that a drug used in medicine has horrific consequences for some does not necessarily mean that such drugs should be banned. It does mean that the potential for such misuse must always be evaluated and actively managed at multiple levels—from federal and state regulations governing the drug's availability to the physician's decision to prescribe or not prescribe the drug to a particular patient.

As for the future of psychoactive drug consumption, much of what has been will be. But there is a danger in seeing all such consumption in terms of a resurfacing of past cycles. Such a view could blind us to that which is fundamentally new, and there are bold breaks from these historical cycles. We have seen in our brief discussion of "T's and Blues" that two drugs with low addiction potential can be combined to form a mixture with a high potential for addiction. This strategic synergism is likely to increase in the future and will pose significant challenges to how we study drugs in medicine and how we regulate access to drugs in the larger society.

We have also seen that slight molecular modifications of a drug can generate profoundly different effects. There is considerable potential for a designer drug disaster within the American illicit drug culture in the coming century. The worst scenario would be the creation of a new designer drug whose short-term euphorigenic effects masked devastating effects revealed only months or years following exposure.

Another principle worth noting is that our knowledge of a drug must be re-evaluated if we change the characteristics of those who consume it. Two trends are noteworthy: the lowered age of regular onset of substance use in America and the increase in late-onset substance use disorders. The trend toward significant pre-adolescent drug experimentation and increased psychoactive drug consumption among seniors with ever-increasing longevity may force a re-evaluation of the effects and dependence potential of certain drugs.

As a people, we will continue, individually and collectively, to seek introspection, stimulation, and anesthesia, and our appetite for particular drugs will shift as our desire for particular types of experiences shift. New drugs that enhance performance and amplify experience will mark a third pharmacological revolution (the earlier eras having been marked by relief from physical and emotional pain and the quest for pleasure). In the enduring search for relief, pleasure, and improvement within the human condition, the line between medicine and intoxicant will remain a thin one. OxyContin is not the first or the last drug that will straddle this line.

Addiction As a Family Disease

Stephanie Brown, Ph.D.

"I'm not hurting anyone. Leave me alone. I can't bear the pain and it's not getting any better. What do you want me to do? Hurt all the time? You probably think I'm making it up."

These are the words of Josh, the twenty-six-year-old son of Maggie and Ted Branton. Josh broke his ribs and injured his back during a football game three years ago. Since then, he's had three surgeries, which have helped correct the damage but have not eliminated the pain. Josh has been living with chronic pain ever since he took that hard hit while scoring the winning touchdown.

Josh has not been able to work and has been living with his parents during his recuperation. He suffers from depression and anxiety as well as chronic pain. He wonders if he'll ever lead a normal life and rages at his parents for their concern about his use of pain medication. Their worry escalated when Josh could not stop taking his medication two months after his last surgery.

Josh takes OxyContin every day. He takes it when he gets up and he takes it throughout the day. He has tried to cut back several times over the last three years, but he says the pain is unbearable. His parents worry constantly that he is taking too much medication, yet they feel guilty about questioning him. They try not to mention it, and they try not to see it. They tell themselves and their friends that Josh is depressed and that he needs his medication just to function. They don't want him to hurt, but they also feel like they've lost the son they used to know. They know that if they say too much to Josh, the fighting starts.

What is the problem here? You may recognize it immediately. You know that Josh is addicted to this drug. He has to have it, even though he firmly believes he doesn't have to have it. You may also see that his parents are deeply involved in Josh's addiction as well. That is, they're part of what has become a family disease. The medication that is supposed to help Josh manage his physical pain has become the center of a new kind of pain: the pain of family addiction. No one knows what to do about this difficult dilemma. The whole family is stuck in a downward spiral of worry, efforts to control what can't be controlled, and increasing anger and resentment. They all know that something is terribly wrong, but no one can say exactly what it is. This family has become organized around Josh's addiction and everyone's efforts to deny that reality while they go on living with it at the same time. This is why addiction is called a family disease.

Addiction As a Family Disease

Earlier chapters in this book have discussed how addiction is a physical, psychological, social, emotional, and spiritual disease characterized by continuous or periodic loss of control. Addiction involves the loss of choice and loss of control over whether, when, or how much of a substance a person has to have. For Josh, it is a loss of control over his need for the drug OxyContin and, eventually, over his behaviors to get it. Addiction also involves a preoccupation with the drug and repeated use of the drug despite adverse consequences. Finally, addiction involves distortions in thinking, particularly denial. Josh feels an intense need for OxyContin, while he maintains that he feels no such need.

An addicted family is the same. As one person, or more, in the family develops an active addiction, everybody else in the family begins to adjust and adapt themselves to the addiction as well. Over time, addiction becomes the central organizing principle for the whole family, shaping family beliefs and influencing everything. The family system becomes distorted, restrictive, and unhealthy as addiction begins to dominate family interactions. There is a big secret, a secret that everybody knows. Worries about the addict's behavior permeate the feelings and motives of everyone in the family, who at the same time deny that there is any problem at all. This is a double-bind that leads to increasingly serious problems for each person in the family and for the family as a whole.

The Branton family is caught in the catch-22 family system that has developed in response to Josh's addiction to OxyContin. Initially, no one questioned Josh's need for medication. And no one noticed when refills became more frequent. Everyone wants Josh to be comfortable, and he is, as long as he can take his meds. From the beginning, everyone knew there would be more surgeries, so no one has pressured Josh back to work or a normal life. He feels continuous pain, so no one questions his continuing use of the medication. The prescription says to take "as needed," so Josh takes it all the time.

Josh has slipped into a physical and emotional dependence on this drug. He's not sure when he became hooked, but his crossover into addiction was quick and intense. He is frightened of the pain and frightened to be without the medication. His parents feel exactly the same. They can't stand to see their son in pain, but they don't know that Josh now needs the medication beyond its prescribed use. Almost imperceptibly, the entire family has adapted their behavior to support Josh's addiction.

Family Addiction As a Developmental Process

An individual's addiction can develop rapidly, as it did for Josh, or very slowly. It can also happen quickly or slowly for the family. Whichever pace, fast or slow, becoming an addicted family is a developmental process and most people don't know it's happening until they're well along the way.

Development usually means "forward growth," a process that builds in layers and stages. Healthy individuals, couples, and families all grow in this forward-moving way. Addiction is a similar developmental process, except movement is backward rather than forward, and growth is restrictive rather than expansive. The process of becoming addicted to a substance, in this case OxyContin, interferes with forward, healthy growth and even stops other kinds of normal development. This shift backward happens first for the addicted individual. Then the entire family joins in.

The backward development of addiction involves an increasing loss of control for the individual and for everyone else. The addicted person has lost control of his or her use of the substance. Josh has become dependent on OxyContin to ease his physical pain. Initially, the drug did just that. It helped. But then his drug turned on him. Josh began to feel a painful need—a combination of physical pain and emotional craving. Once he acts on his feeling of need, he can't stop. He needs more and more OxyContin just to feel numb. Josh now panics every time he needs a refill. Will someone deny him his pills? Josh no longer has a choice about whether or when he takes his medication. He has to have it all the time. He has lost control.

It's hard to grasp the fact that, in addition to the addict losing control, family members have lost control too. They cannot control the addicted person, and they cannot control, stop, or reverse the downward path into illness and unhealthy family functioning that is now underway. Everyone thinks that all will be well if they can just figure out how to get the addict to stop. Family members often invest all their energy into trying to control the addict. But no one can get this person to stop. Worst of all, they can't see that they, too, are developing their own addictive behaviors, thoughts, and feelings.

It is particularly hard for families to recognize addiction when the substance is a prescribed medication. How is the family supposed to know what is best for the patient? How can anyone expect the addicted person to do without medicine? So these families often get caught in the trap of trying to get the addicted person to cut back, to "get this thing under control." In an addicted family, everyone is trying to get control of someone or something that can't be controlled. Being in an addicted family is like trying to go up the down escalator.

The Turn toward Addiction

Early in his recuperation, Josh makes a turn toward addiction. He begins to need OxyContin for more than the treatment of his physical pain. He has no idea that he has developed an emotional dependence. It just seems to him that he doesn't want to hurt. It isn't until a few years after his treatment for addiction that Josh is able to reconstruct the turn he made into addiction. Josh remembers the pain he felt on the playing field. He was hurt badly, and he knew he wouldn't play football again for a long time. The paramedics gave him pain medication immediately, and he relaxed. He never forgot that feeling of instant internal quiet, instant soothing.

Immediately after his surgery, Josh asked for more pain medication. He had made his turn. From that point on, he changed his thinking in order to reassure himself and his parents that he was fine, that he was only taking his medication as prescribed, and that he would soon be healed and off of this substance anyway. "This is temporary," he told them, even though he already knew he loved this medicine.

The family makes this same turn toward addiction. It just comes later, in response to the presence of an active addict in the family. The family's turn toward addiction is a turn toward deception, a turn toward distortion in logic and explanation. The family, supporting Josh, bands together, usually without any awareness at all, to deny his addiction and support his use of OxyContin. At the same time, Josh's parents harbor secret concerns: Josh takes way too much OxyContin, way too often, and seems to be a very different person much of the time.

As addiction progresses, family members need to distort more and more of what they see, hear, feel, and know to be reality. They quiet their worries with new explanations. Josh's parents keep saying, "What do we know? He must need this medication. How can we outguess the doctors? How can we take away the medicine that relieves his pain?"

Josh's parents don't know that he is copying prescriptions, stealing money from them, and visiting several doctors in several towns to refill his medicines. This massive deception works for a long time to keep his parents from articulating their growing concerns. They feel guilty for lacking compassion, and they are afraid to question him. They wonder if they are to blame for Josh's increasingly angry, withdrawn, and secretive behavior. They wonder what they have done wrong to cause this.

This is the family disease, like a virus or a cancer. As addiction progresses, all family members sacrifice their perceptions and explanations of reality, and their honesty with themselves and others. They succumb to the growing infection organized by this now-pathological family system.

Trouble on Every Front

Addiction inevitably begins to dominate every aspect of family life. As the family system grows more distressed, the home environment becomes increasingly tense and constricted. The environment holds the emotion of all that's happening in the family. Even outsiders can sense the chaos, confusion, mistrust, loneliness, and isolation as family members struggle to cope with a reality that can't be fixed. This kind of environment becomes a trauma in its own right. This underlying fear holds a family in its grips.

The individual who lives in this trauma gets lost, submerged in the increasingly distorted and defended swamp of false reality. Family members do the same thing: Each individual loses himself or herself to the disease of addiction. All individuals—parents, spouses, and children—lose their sense of reality. Individuals sacrifice themselves to preserve this unhealthy family system. As they give up their own view of the world, they adapt themselves to a pathology that protects the big family secret. Addiction becomes the new organizing principle of family dynamics.

The Family System

Family systems theory started in the 1950s and 1960s as a way of thinking about how parts relate to a whole. Family systems theorists, such as Gregory Bateson, Murray Bowen, and Salvador Minuchin, described how families or other organized units work. All families have certain mechanisms and structures—like schedules, for example—that allow them to function. All families have certain relationship and behavior patterns of interaction—like parenting roles, for example—that maintain a family's sense of balance, or what's technically called *homeostasis*. Ultimately, all groups or families strive to find and maintain stability, consistency, and cohesion.

Now throw addiction into the mix, and family balance begins to shift. The shifting and wavering may be subtle at first. Nobody blows the whistle because people usually can't see what's happening. By the time they finally do realize what is going on, they're afraid that blowing the whistle will only upset the balance even more.

As Dr. Drew Pinsky discussed in chapter 1, the need for a sense of connection with others, what is called *attachment*, drives people to go along with the family dynamics. As we can see with Josh, his parents suspect he is in trouble, but they are afraid to name the reality. It's as if speaking up will make things even worse. So they don't speak, and eventually their vision becomes even more clouded.

So the family makes room for this new intruder: addiction. The family becomes less flexible, more rigid. The family, subtly or quite overtly, changes its rules, roles, rituals, hierarchies, and boundaries as it tightens up.

Rules

Family rules guide what happens in every family and influence every family's stability and identity. For example, a family rule might be "We are private people, so we don't talk about personal things." This is why, in Reesa's family, it has taken four years for anyone to note that Reesa is asleep every afternoon by 3:00, awake again by 5:00, and nodding off at 7:00. Reesa, a wife and mother of young children, is in a constant state of near-coma, yet everyone says she just needs a lot of sleep.

Reesa got hooked on OxyContin following a complicated dental surgery. When her dental problems healed, she developed back and neck pain, and then muscle spasms. She was diagnosed with a nerve disorder that was the cause of chronic pain, and she was given a convenient, refillable prescription for OxyContin to take "as needed."

So here we go again. Reesa's family has adapted itself to her illnesses and her increasing debilitation. She is a wife and mother with chronic illness. Everyone follows the rule not to talk about anything so personal. They have also changed other rules. It used to be that everyone had chores, everyone showed up for meals on time, and Reesa was the organizer.

Now, the family members accommodate Reesa's addiction. She doesn't do her own chores anymore, she sometimes doesn't start dinner, and she doesn't show up to sit at the table during meals. So, other family members fill in and take up the slack. They tiptoe around so as not to disturb her. After going through treatment for her drug addiction, Reesa told her family how awful it felt to be so ignored during that time. They were just trying to help, just trying to ease her worry. Becoming an exception to her family's rules slowed Reesa down in getting help.

Roles

Roles are the functions performed by each person in a family or group. Roles can be useful or not useful, healthy or not healthy. Roles are essential to any family system or any relationship. Knowing who we are and what we're supposed to do in a given situation gives each of us a sense of value.

In a healthy family, someone has the role of breadwinner, someone plans the meals, and someone does the laundry. Everybody may do all these things, but each person in the family knows who's in charge of what, and things work. There are also emotional roles. Mom might be the "emotional rod," the one who has the feeling first and who encourages feelings in others. Dad might be the disciplinarian, or vice versa. It works, even if people sometimes wish Mom could be a little clearer about holding limits, and that Dad could just have a feeling every now and then.

As addiction develops, roles can become confused, distorted, or reassigned. People will also adapt new roles, including ways to maintain the family's denial, while trying to solve the problem too. These roles were spelled out many years ago in relation to children raised by alcoholic parents.[1] These kids become the "hero," the "caretaker," the "placater," the "comic," the "act-outer," or all of the above, in an effort to cope with an uncopeable situation: their parents' out-of-control drinking.

During Reesa's active addiction, her kids learn to get themselves up in the morning, to be extra quiet, and to take over all the organizing jobs of their mother. They all begin to view Reesa as the child, the one who needs protection and quiet. They think of themselves as parents, working to keep the family running. This role reversal happens all the time in addicted families.

Rituals

Rituals are established customs that help define a family and provide an emotional bond. Healthy rituals are very much part of a family's healthy identity, and they contribute to cohesiveness. Unhealthy rituals work the same way, but they tend to reinforce family pathology.

Reesa's family used to celebrate each person's birthday with a special dinner and a family evening of board games. Everybody in this family was a top-notch Monopoly player. As Reesa developed her addiction to OxyContin, she stopped joining the games. Eventually she stopped preparing the party dinners, and then she forgot the birthdays. Everybody said they really didn't care, but it was sad when Ginny, the youngest, wrote her mother a note, reminding her, "It's my eleventh birthday in a few days, and wouldn't it be nice to have a party?"

Hierarchies and Boundaries

These are the ladders and the fences of family life. Hierarchy refers to levels of power. The person at the top of the hierarchy is the one who's in charge, the one who sets the rules, roles, and rituals in the family. The boundaries keep the family together. Sometimes family boundaries are super loose, so there's a lot of confusion, a lot of coming and going that works. It might get pretty chaotic, but it's okay. Other families have a tighter "sense of fence." It's harder for people to come and go within the family and harder for visitors to feel like insiders.

There's a big range of normal, of course. Healthy families develop their own ways, and they work. But addiction disrupts the usual hierarchies and the boundaries. The person in charge may also be the most impaired, which becomes a major disruption. Or, the person in charge may no longer be in charge—someone else steps in, as in Reesa's case. The family used to have a lot of company, but now no one comes over to visit. One time an old friend dropped in and that was the last of the drop-ins. From then on, people were screened at the front door. They were screened on the phone. Nobody could crash this fortress anymore. That left Reesa even more isolated and the family more closed in.

An addicted family system stays shut down because family communications become distorted. People know they can't talk about what is real. Communication becomes indirect, even dominated by a new code. Reesa's husband and kids refer to their mother's "condition." Josh's family members talk about his stress and anxiety, his "situation."

Contrary to popular thinking, the addicted family is a "functional system." It works. In fact, people go to great lengths to keep it working, twisting themselves into pretzels to adapt to the pathology of addiction. So, yes, the system works. But it's mighty unhealthy. As the family gets stretched to the breaking point, the system begins to crack. It becomes dysfunctional because now it doesn't work. Unfortunately, it's hard for families to change. And a dysfunctional system can endure for a long time.

The Environment

Bad things often appear first in a family's emotional environment. This is the context of family life, the "atmosphere" or the "feel" of things. It's the mood, the tone, the kind and degree of chaos, and whether there is physical and emotional safety. This is where the tension breeds, where the anger and resentment settle in. This is the dark mood that hits like a storm when Josh's mother suggests he try to decrease his medication and he starts screaming.

The environment holds the trauma of powerlessness, the emotions of being out of control. The environment, no matter how organized and tightly controlled, becomes chaotic because the core of the family is now out of control. Things become inconsistent, unpredictable. Nobody has any sense of trust that things aren't going to fall apart. So everybody watches. Everybody goes on guard to ward off the inevitable bad things that will start to happen.

Early on, Josh's mother feels the effects of the trauma of the family addiction. She can't sleep at night as she worries about what is happening to her son. But that scares her so much that she convinces herself that he doesn't have a problem. She decides that she has the problem instead. She creates different scenarios about what is really wrong, each drama ending up with her to blame. She should have supported Josh more in his fights with his father when Josh was a teenager. She should have set firmer limits for Josh and his younger sister, Kendra, when they were fighting. She should not have looked the other way when Josh and his friends were smoking pot in the backyard a few years ago. By the second year of Josh's "recuperation," his mother has a prescription for sleeping pills and anxiety medication, both addictive substances.

Josh's father also develops scenarios of failure. He should have played more with both of his kids, but he was working hard, so how could he? Josh's father ends up agreeing with his wife that she is to blame, and he begins to point out how she has failed them all throughout the kids' childhood.

Josh's parents begin to argue frequently. While they are both angry at Josh for using too much medication, they reason that Josh's injury is not his fault. So they yell at each other instead. The mood at home is one of brooding tension and hostility.

The environment in Reesa's family is more subdued. There is an almost palpable feeling of grief, of something really wrong here, but no one can name it. The kids miss their mother, and they need her. They are scared about what is happening as she drops out of sight for hours and then for days at a time. Members of this family feel physically safe; they don't think anyone will blow up. But they feel scared, lost, and lonely.

Luckily, Reesa and her family find help. At a routine appointment, Reesa's husband tells his physician that he has been having trouble sleeping. His doctor wants to know more. The story dribbles out and then it pours. Alarmed, the doctor immediately intervenes, bringing Reesa in for a consultation, working with the doctors who have been treating her and pre-scribing OxyContin, and referring her for addiction treatment. This is a hard process. Everyone is scared, but Reesa goes to treatment, gets off the drug, and gets well. It takes a long time, and there are a lot of scars for everyone.

Individual Development

By the time the family disease is well underway, each family member has sacrificed his or her individual health, well-being, personality, and unique character. Each family member's good qualities are lost or covered up as distortions and defenses dominate the family system.

This is a loss of self. This is what's been called codepen-dence. Individuals give up their real selves, that rock-solid sense of "who I am," that capacity to see, feel, think, and say what is what. Of course, many people struggle to be real anyway, even without addiction. There are plenty of pressures in relationships and in society to inhibit people from being themselves.

But with addiction, people slowly but surely slip into what is called a "false self." This is the facade of denial that main-tains "nothing is wrong here." This mask exists to preserve the family's unhealthy, precarious balance. People come to know deep down that they must submerge their healthy selves, the person who does know what's going on, in order to prevent calamity. Yet, it's this giving up of the self that further protects the downward spiral of addiction.

Codependence is the automatic sacrifice of self to the

pathology of addiction. It's the agreement to collude with the addiction. It's the willingness to bury the self in favor of maintaining an unhealthy relationship or family system. Adults have a choice about this, even though they often don't know it. Kids, especially young kids, don't have a choice. The younger they are, the more their normal development will be skewed by the family's turn toward addiction. During Reesa's active addiction, Ginny tried to get her mother to be a mother, but it didn't work.

Ginny told herself that she must be a bad daughter, that she must not deserve a birthday party, because her mother had forgotten her important day. Ginny couldn't grasp that her mother was ill, that her mother was powerless over her addiction to OxyContin.

As addiction becomes the most powerful dynamic in a family, individuals may balk as the tide turns toward pathology. They may even mention the word "OxyContin" early on and express a worry that there's just too much of it being used. But in most families, this freedom to name the pathology won't continue. It stirs things up too much to tell the truth. So, usually, people stop talking and begin the process of distortion and defense.

We can see this with Josh and his family. After his football injury, Josh comes to think of himself as disabled. In the beginning, he thought it would be temporary and he was optimistic about the future. He thought about returning to the work world and playing soccer instead of football. As one year turned into two years, then three years, Josh lost his sense of a hopeful future. So have his parents. They make plans to turn the family room into a sick room, or what they call the "recoup room."

Josh's parents quit their evening bridge group and book

clubs. Their strong sense of themselves as Maggie Branton and Ted Branton fades. They are now the parents of an invalid. They have no idea they are the parents of an addict, that they are now part of this disabling disease.

Defenses

Family members living with addiction make a pact with denial. Denial says, "It isn't so." That statement becomes the central organizing principle for the family and the first sentence in the family's new identity of "who we are."

Denial operates on every level. Denial requires changes in thinking. People start to rationalize why the addiction that is really happening isn't happening. Maggie and Ted keep telling themselves that doctors know best, and besides, Josh's problems are probably due to the fact that they are bad parents. Then they bring in the evidence to prove that they have messed up badly.

Here is another astonishing quality of a family living with addiction: We can't have feelings about a reality that is not supposed to exist. So all the feelings that dominate the environment—the fear, anxiety, anger, sorrow—are denied, expressed as something else, or channeled into new illnesses. Maggie becomes depressed and anxious, and she can't sleep—all understandable reactions to living with the trauma of addiction.

Denial requires more and more distortion. Then it requires greater efforts at control to keep it intact. This need for control becomes the organizing principle for each person. This drive for control becomes a frenzy for many, a ratcheting up of behaviors to make things okay, making it even harder to see that it all started to protect an addiction. Now everybody is addicted.

Control is an issue for everybody, even in a family where no addiction exists. Feeling "in control" or feeling "out of control" is part of being human. Negotiating control is a central feature of all relationships, but when addiction is the organizing feature in a family, the feelings of loss of control and profound helplessness permeate everything. In fact, this trauma is the result of this magnitude of loss of control.

Recovery

The good news is that people living with a high degree of addiction-related trauma can find a way "out." Yes, people recover.[2] Families do face the reality of what they've denied, and addicts stop using the OxyContin or other addictive substances.

You may think that recovery simply means the addict stops using the drug and everybody goes back to normal. If addiction to the drug OxyContin is quick, and the process of becoming an addicted individual and an addicted family is brief, the individual and the family may indeed go back to normal. But this kind of experience with addiction is rare. That's because becoming addicted is so insidious. Everybody becomes lost in the pathology before they know what's wrong.

Most addicts and their families will experience a *process* of recovery, in addition to the *event* of becoming abstinent. All the adjustments they made to becoming addicted will not just disappear overnight. Some families will have to grow into a healthy family, perhaps for the first time. Others will have to work hard on repairing the healthy boundaries they once had. Getting to recovery and being in recovery are almost like a mirror image of the downward spiral of addiction. Most families will make a turn toward abstinence, just like they turned toward addiction. Then they begin a developmental process of new growth, this time moving away from addiction in their behavior, thinking, feeling, and patterns of relating. If the family has reached out for help, and if one or more members of the family belong to a Twelve Step program, it's possible that no one will go back to the old way.

In recovery, individuals grow into a new sense of self, and the family will develop a new sense of themselves in relation to others. Step-by-step, everybody in the family will move from denial to telling the truth; each person will move from a false self to a real self, as they connect the dots of what really happened. The recent past of horrendous addiction comes into focus. No one can believe they couldn't see it, and no one can believe they could have gotten into such trouble. Now it seems so clear.

This glance at reality can be a sharp, stinging jolt, or a subtle, gradual coming into focus. Reesa's husband, Barak, began to think that she was using too much OxyContin. He talked with his physician, and intervention and treatment followed. There was no jolt. Just a steady progression of getting clear.

In Josh's family, it happens with a jolt. After three years, Josh's mom "hits bottom." In desperation, she talks with her rabbi about how sad and frightened she is, and describes the family's growing isolation. The rabbi sighs and gently tells her that she is living with addiction. He sees it and he names it.

At first, the word *addiction* strikes at Maggie like a knife. She is quiet. Then she knows. She is sad at first, but she also feels relief. Her rabbi gives her the name of a counselor and she calls that afternoon.

Maggie starts to look, to see, and to say out loud what she is seeing. There is more fighting than usual, but she sticks to her guns. Ted goes to therapy with her too. They invite Josh to talk about family addiction. He refuses at first, and then he agrees.

After several difficult months, the Branton family makes their turn away from active addiction. Maggie goes to Nar-Anon, a Twelve Step program for family members of people addicted to drugs and Ted follows. Eventually, Josh talks with his doctors and embarks on a plan to withdraw from OxyContin.

When he is just about off of the drug, he panics. What will he do if he feels too much pain? So he ups his medication again. Finally, he starts therapy, goes to Narcotics Anonymous (NA), and gets clean. Is this a happy ending? No, but it is the beginning of a new process of family growth.

The Developmental Process of Recovery

As the family moves forward, changes begin to occur in the family system, the environment, and for each individual. Now, instead of being organized around the pathology of addiction, the family reorganizes around recovery. Initially, they haven't a clue what this means, but they will learn.

It's critical to reach out to a pastor, a rabbi, a therapist, a doctor, a friend, or a member of a Twelve Step program for help. These resources can help family members

- articulate their stories of how addiction affected them
- finally feel the pain of living with active addiction
- start to change destructive behaviors

Family recovery is especially hard because everybody thinks that it should be easy. Family members think they'll go back to normal once the addiction is named and the addict gets clean. A lot does get better, and it's a relief to know what was wrong. But it's a shock when former "normal" behaviors don't work anymore. Nobody wants to hear that they all have work to do.

The Family System

In some families, the "pre-addiction" system worked and it was healthy. So, if the addiction was brief, the family reverts to this system. But most families find that they can't go back. They got too messed up being an addicted family. Then they recognize, as they try out the old rules, roles, and rituals, that they weren't so healthy after all. So, many families come to see that they were headed for addiction no matter what. Now they have an opportunity to start over, to look at themselves as a family that lost control. What do they have to change so they don't get into this kind of trouble again?

Initially, in recovery, the focus is on the individuals and not on the system. Growth starts for the individuals who separate from the pathology of the addicted system. Sometimes this goes smoothly, as each person in the family recognizes the reality of addiction and accepts help. As the addictive system loses its power, it doesn't work anymore to pull people back into pathology. But sometimes only one person breaks denial and steps out of the system. Others resist. This usually creates an even more hostile environment.

Josh, Maggie, and Ted all move into recovery. They focus on their individual growth and soon start talking together about what happened. They all support each other in standing firm. Reesa also goes into recovery. Her husband supports her but does not see that he has anything to change. He waits for her to return to how she used to be. The kids are upset because, yes, their mother is awake now, but she is edgy and frequently gone at recovery meetings. Everybody wants Mom to be home and to be "mothering." Yet Reesa needs to focus on early abstinence. Her family struggles for a long time.

It's a shocking paradox: The family system, so powerful in its support of addiction, collapses into an undefined system.

The family goes from total absorption in the disturbed system to no system at all. People flounder and go back to old ways. It's difficult to hang on and trust that a new, healthy system will grow on a foundation of healthy individual development.

The Environment
Some aspects of the family environment change quickly. For example, the danger, anger, and hopelessness that permeated the atmosphere diminish. People often feel safer physically and slightly safer emotionally once family members are talking about the addiction and what really happened. But the environment remains uncertain, tense, and anxiety ridden. The trauma of addiction leaves the family with many undefined unknowns about recovery and fears of relapse. People are wary. They wonder, "Is this recovery going to last? How can we trust each other?"

Maggie and Ted start going to Nar-Anon and continue their counseling. They struggle over lots of issues. They don't want to leave Josh alone, and it is hard to stop nagging him about going to recovery meetings. They need to shift their worries from him to themselves. This shift to focus on themselves will help interrupt the unhealthy family system, yet neither Maggie nor Ted know how to look at themselves. So, for a time, the absence of the former family system causes more anxiety for everyone. They all feel like they are fumbling around as the mood shifts from terrified and raging to cautious and careful.

Over time, the environment will calm down, helped by new rules, roles, and rituals that develop to support the early work of recovery. Sometimes this is as simple as keeping a calendar on the fridge to track everybody's whereabouts. People learn how to work on their own, and how to work together, in the absence of a healthy family system. The environment begins to reflect the healthy growth of each person.

In early recovery, Maggie, Ted, and Josh agree not to talk about anything except the weather and what is for dinner. After a few months, you begin to hear occasional laughter. Then one day, they start talking with each other about their programs of recovery. Now, they feel safe enough to share with each other what they are learning. They are careful not to go too fast. They return to their family counselor for help with opening up more painful memories.

Over several years, the Branton family grows into a solid, healthy recovering family. The atmosphere is warm and supportive. This is not a return to the same old happy family. Rather, this is a new way of relating. They have never felt this easy with each other. Their daughter, Kendra, away at college during most of Josh's active addiction, joins in readily when she returns home after graduation. She loves the changes everyone is making. She has lots to say about her own child-hood, and she knows she has lots to look at in herself too.

The environment in Reesa's family also stays tense for a long time. She grows in recovery but always has a sense that her family would be happier if she could go back home, be the "old" Reesa, and take care of all of them. She imagines them saying, "Can't you be the same? Just don't take OxyContin."

No, Reesa can't be the same. She's been addicted to OxyContin for a long time. In recovery, she begins to realize that before the pain medication, she'd been taking daily tranquilizers and uppers. She's been addicted for a long time, and she has a lot of emotional work to do. At home, she feels vulnerable and scared. She feels a pervasive tone of impatience that is hard to ignore.

As the months pass and Reesa grows more secure in her identity as a "recovering addict," the tension in the family quiets. No one else is getting any help, but things are okay. On

Ginny's fourteenth birthday, Reesa throws her a wonderful birthday party. These have been routine again for several years. But this time, Ginny thanks her mother for the party and for being in recovery. Everyone begins to cry. They start remembering how frightened they were. After this, the family grows more open and each person begins to look at himself or herself, just like Reesa has done.

Individual Development

The beginning of recovery for each individual is all about staying abstinent. It's especially hard for family members to see that they were addicted too, and that they have work to do. Many family members want to settle back and wait for the addict to get well, and they don't want to wait too long.

It's hard for family members to see that they got hooked too, and that they need to be in recovery, just like the person who took the OxyContin. Maggie doesn't resist. She is relieved and grateful when her rabbi tells her she is suffering from family addiction. She goes to Nar-Anon immediately and holds tight to her new knowledge. She never wavers.

However, Maggie has a harder time digging into the work of recovery. She needs to look at herself, a "self" she defines by her roles such as *wife, mother,* and *caregiver.* "I take care of others," she says, but she begins to see that there is no Maggie besides her role with others. So she naturally believes that she is to blame for everything. Identifying herself as a family member in recovery will just deepen her guilt.

The hardest part of recovery for Maggie is letting go of worrying about Josh. It was her job to help him, to support him, and now that he is in recovery, she wants to be as good a mother as she can possibly be. How can that mean letting go? How can she be a good mother if all she thinks about is herself?

What a paradox this is. Each person in the family has to grow a new sense of identity.

Barak and the kids resist being in recovery for several years. They are glad Reesa isn't hooked on OxyContin anymore, but the family isn't the same. Reesa has changed a lot, and they are jealous of her recovery meetings. Luckily, over time, they see that she has something they want too. It begins at Ginny's birthday party. From that point on, each person in the family starts his or her own recovery process.

The Long Haul

The recovery process doesn't have a definable ending. Problems occur, and initially, it's hard for the family to know what they're doing or how to solve anything more difficult than what to have for dinner. Yet, they have to deal with serious problems, in the beginning and over time. The family in recovery gets to face life and to show up to deal with everything. They are not magically immune from all the challenges of everyday living.

Growth, however, enables everyone to accept responsibility for themselves, as individuals, and to refuse to accept responsibility for anyone else. In other words, they develop new boundaries that help them say "no" to situations that pulled them into an addictive family system.

Now, both of these families are grateful. It's been about five years for Josh and his family. They have a healthy family system, and Josh is no longer disabled by addiction. Josh moved to his own apartment during his first year of recovery and went back to work. A pain specialist helped him learn to cope with daily pain, without addictive medication.

Reesa and Barak are also in stable recovery. They continue active involvement in their recovery programs. Everyone says they're glad they all got help. At first, it was good to have Mom clean and that was enough. But eventually, it wasn't enough. They could have more and they went for it.

APPENDIX A

PRINCIPLES OF EFFECTIVE TREATMENT

1. **No single treatment is appropriate for all individuals.** Matching treatment settings, interventions, and services to each individual's particular problems and needs is critical to his or her ultimate success in returning to productive functioning in the family, workplace, and society.

2. **Treatment needs to be readily available.** Because individuals who are addicted to drugs may be uncertain about entering treatment, taking advantage of opportunities when they are ready for treatment is crucial. Potential treatment applicants can be lost if treatment is not immediately available or is not readily accessible.

3. **Effective treatment attends to multiple needs of the individual, not just his or her drug use.** To be effective, treatment must address the individual's drug use and any associated medical, psychological, social, vocational, and legal problems.

4. **An individual's treatment and services plan must be assessed continually and modified as necessary to ensure that the plan meets the person's changing needs.** A patient may require varying combinations of services and treatment components during the course of treatment and recovery. In addition to counseling or psychotherapy, a patient at times may require medication, other medical services, family therapy, parenting instruction, vocational

From U.S. Department of Health and Human Services, National Institutes of Health, National Institute on Drug Abuse, *Principles of Drug Addiction Treatment: A Research Based Guide* (printed October 1999, reprinted July 2000), NIH publication no. 00-4180.

rehabilitation, and social and legal services. It is critical that the treatment approach be appropriate to the individual's age, gender, ethnicity, and culture.

5. **Remaining in treatment for an adequate period of time is critical for treatment effectiveness.** The appropriate duration for an individual depends on his or her problems and needs. Research indicates that for most patients, the threshold of significant improvement is reached at about 3 months in treatment. After this threshold is reached, additional treatment can produce further progress toward recovery. Because people often leave treatment prematurely, programs should include strategies to engage and keep patients in treatment.

6. **Counseling (individual and/or group) and other behavioral therapies are critical components of effective treatment for addiction.** In therapy, patients address issues of motivation, build skills to resist drug use, replace drug-using activities with constructive and rewarding nondrug-using activities, and improve problem-solving abilities. Behavioral therapy also facilitates interpersonal relationships and the individual's ability to function in the family and community.

7. **Medications are an important element of treatment for many patients, especially when combined with counseling and other behavioral therapies.** Methadone and levo-alpha-acetylmethadol (LAAM) are very effective in helping individuals addicted to heroin or other opiates stabilize their lives and reduce their illicit drug use. Naltrexone is also an effective medication for some opiate addicts and some patients with co-occurring alcohol dependence. For persons addicted to nicotine, a nicotine replacement product (such as patches or gum) or an oral medication (such as bupropion) can be an effective component of treatment. For patients with mental disorders, both behavioral treatments and medications can be critically important.

8. **Addicted or drug-abusing individuals with coexisting mental disorders should have both disorders treated in an integrated way.** Because addictive disorders and mental disorders often occur in the same individual, patients presenting for either condition should be assessed and treated for the co-occurrence of the other type of disorder.

9. **Medical detoxification is only the first stage of addiction treatment and by itself does little to change long-term drug use.** Medical detoxification safely manages the acute physical symptoms of withdrawal associated with stopping drug use. While detoxification alone is rarely sufficient to help addicts achieve long-term abstinence, for some individuals it is a strongly indicated precursor to effective drug addiction treatment.

10. **Treatment does not need to be voluntary to be effective.** Strong motivation can facilitate the treatment process. Sanctions or enticements in the family, employment setting, or criminal justice system can increase significantly both treatment entry and retention rates and the success of drug treatment interventions.

11. **Possible drug use during treatment must be monitored continuously.** Lapses to drug use can occur during treatment. The objective monitoring of a patient's drug and alcohol use during treatment, such as through urinalysis or other tests, can help the patient withstand urges to use drugs. Such monitoring also can provide early evidence of drug use so that the individual's treatment plan can be adjusted. Feedback to patients who test positive for illicit drug use is an important element of monitoring.

12. **Treatment programs should provide assessment for HIV/AIDS, hepatitis B and C, tuberculosis and other infectious diseases, and counseling to help patients modify or change behaviors that place themselves or others at risk of infection.** Counseling can help patients avoid high-risk behavior. Counseling also can help people who are already infected manage their illness.

13. **Recovery from drug addiction can be a long-term process and frequently requires multiple episodes of treatment.** As with other chronic illnesses, relapses to drug use can occur during or after successful treatment episodes. Addicted individuals may require prolonged treatment and multiple episodes of treatment to achieve long-term abstinence and fully restored functioning. Participation in self-help support programs during and following treatment often is helpful in maintaining abstinence.

THE TWELVE STEPS OF ALCOHOLICS ANONYMOUS

1. We admitted we were powerless over alcohol—that our lives had become unmanageable.
2. Came to believe that a Power greater than ourselves could restore us to sanity.
3. Made a decision to turn our will and our lives over to the care of God *as we understood Him.*
4. Made a searching and fearless moral inventory of ourselves.
5. Admitted to God, to ourselves, and to another human being the exact nature of our wrongs.
6. Were entirely ready to have God remove all these defects of character.
7. Humbly asked Him to remove our shortcomings.
8. Made a list of all persons we had harmed, and became willing to make amends to them all.
9. Made direct amends to such people wherever possible, except when to do so would injure them or others.
10. Continued to take personal inventory and when we were wrong promptly admitted it.
11. Sought through prayer and meditation to improve our conscious contact with God *as we understood Him,* praying only for knowledge of His will for us and the power to carry that out.
12. Having had a spiritual awakening as the result of these steps, we tried to carry this message to alcoholics, and to practice these principles in all our affairs.

From *Alcoholics Anonymous,* 4th ed. (New York: Alcoholics Anonymous World Services, Inc., 2001), 59–60.

NOTES

Chapter 1:
OxyContin and Other Prescription Pain Medication

1. See opioids.com/oxycodone/oxycontin.htm.

2. Ibid.

3. Ibid.

4. Ibid.

5. For further reading on this topic, please see the following: Allan N. Schore, *Affect Regulation and the Repair of the Self* (New York: W. W. Norton & Company, 2003) and Allan N. Schore, *Affect Regulation and the Origin of the Self: The Neurobiology of Emotional Development* (Mahwah, N.J.: Lawrence Erlbaum Associates, Inc., 1999).

6. See www.aapainmanage.org.

7. Ibid.

8. Ibid.

9. Ibid.

10. Peter Fonagy, György Gergely, Elliot L. Jurist, and Mary Target, *Affect Regulation, Mentalization, and the Development of Self* (New York: Other Press, 2002).

11. Ibid.

Chapter 2: How Addiction Treatment Works

1. Alan I. Leshner, "Understanding Drug Addiction: Insights from the Research," in *Principles of Addiction Medicine,* 3d ed., ed. Allan W. Graham, Terry K. Schultz, Michael F. Mayo-Smith, Richard K. Ries, and Bonnie B. Wilford (Chevy Chase, Md.: American Society of Addiction Medicine, 2003).

2. D. C. Lewis, "A Disease Model of Addiction," in *Principles of Addiction Medicine,* ed. Norman S. Miller and Martin C. Doot (Chevy Chase, Md.: American Society of Addiction Medicine, 1994), 1–7.

3. U.S. Department of Health and Human Services, Substance Abuse and Mental Health Services Administration, *SAMHSA National Survey of Substance Abuse Treatment Services* (2000), available at www.samhsa.gov.

4. Henry R. Kranzler and Jerome H. Jaffe, "Pharmacologic Interventions for Alcoholism," in *Principles of Addiction Medicine,* 3d ed., ed. Allan W. Graham, Terry K. Schultz, Michael F. Mayo-Smith, Richard K. Ries, and Bonnie B. Wilford (Chevy Chase, Md.: American Society of Addiction Medicine, 2003).

5. W. A. Hunt, L. W. Barnett, and L. G. Branch, "Relapse Rates in Addiction Programs," *Journal of Clinical Psychology* 27, no. 4 (1971): 455–56.

6. J. Morgenstern, E. Labouvie, B. S. McCrady, C. W. Kahler, and R. M. Frey, "Affiliation with Alcoholics Anonymous after Treatment: A Study of Its Therapeutic Effects and Mechanisms of Action," *Journal of Consulting and Clinical Psychology* 65, no. 5 (1997): 768–77.

7. J. S. Gavaler, "Sex-Related Differences in Ethanol-Induced Liver Disease: Artificial or Not?" *Alcoholism: Clinical and Experimental Research* 6, no. 2 (1982): 186–96.

8. A. Urbano-Marquez, R. Estruch, J. Fernandez-Sola, J. M. Nicolas, J. C. Pare, and E. Rubin, "The Greater Risk of Alcoholic Cardiomyopathy and Myopathy in Women Compared with Men," *Journal of the American Medical Association* 274, no. 2 (1995): 149–54.

9. K. Mann, A. Batra, A. Grunthner, and G. Schroth, "Do Women Develop Alcoholic Brain Damage More Readily Than Men?" *Alcoholism: Clinical and Experimental Research* 16, no. 6 (1992): 1052–56.

10. H. M. Pettinati, J. D. Pierce, A. L. Wolf, M. R. Rukstalis, and C. P. O'Brien, "Gender Difference in Comorbidly Depressed Alcohol-Dependent Outpatients," *Alcoholism: Clinical and Experimental Research* 21, no. 9 (1997): 1742–46.

11. S. A. Brown and M. A. Schuckit, "Changes in Depression among Abstinent Alcoholics," *Journal of Studies on Alcohol* 49, no. 5 (1988): 412–17.

12. J. H. Shore, "The Oregon Experience with Impaired Physicians on Probation: An Eight-Year Follow-Up," *Journal of the American Medical Association* 257, no. 21 (1987): 2931–34.

13. A. T. McLellan, D. C. Lewis, C. P. O'Brien, and H. D. Kleber, "Drug Dependence, a Chronic Medical Illness: Implications for Treatment, Insurance, and Outcomes Evaluation," *Journal of the American Medical Association* 284, no. 13 (2000): 1689–95.

14. R. L. Hubbard, S. G. Craddock, P. M. Flynn, J. Anderson, and R. M. Etheridge, "Overview of One-Year Follow-Up Outcomes in the Drug Abuse Treatment Outcome Study (DATOS)," *Psychology of Addictive Behaviors* 11, no. 4 (1997): 261–78.

Chapter 3: How to Intervene on a Loved One's Addiction

1. A complete description of CRAFT can be found in Robert J. Meyers and Brenda L. Wolfe, *Get Your Loved One Sober: Alternatives to Nagging, Pleading, and Threatening* (Center City, Minn.: Hazelden, 2004).

2. R. J. Meyers, W. R. Miller, J. E. Smith, and J. S. Tonigan, "A Randomized Trial of Two Methods for Engaging Treatment-Refusing Drug Users through Concerned Significant Others," *Journal of Consulting and Clinical Psychology* 70, no. 5 (2002): 1182–85. W. R. Miller, R. J. Meyers, and J. S. Tonigan, "Engaging the Unmotivated in Treatment for Alcohol Problems: A Comparison of Three Strategies for Intervention through Family Members," *Journal of Consulting and Clinical Psychology* 67, no. 5 (1999): 688–97.

3. Miller, Meyers, Tonigan, "Engaging the Unmotivated in Treatment for Alcohol Problems."

4. See Meyers and Wolfe, *Get Your Loved One Sober.*

Chapter 4: OxyContin Addiction

1. L. Skrebowski, "Oxycodone Explained," Guardian Unlimited (24 March 2002), available at observer.guardian.co.uk/uk_news/story/0,6903,673228,00.html.

2. U.S. Department of Health and Human Services, Substance Abuse and Mental Health Services Administration, Office of Applied Studies, *The DASIS Report: Treatment Admissions Involving Narcotic Painkillers* (26 December 2003), available at www.oas.samhsa.gov/2k3/PainTX/ PainTX.cfm.

3. J. Young, "Patent Medicines: The Early Post-frontier Phase," *Journal of the Illinois State Historical Society* 46 (1953): 254–64.

4. J. Young, *The Toadstool Millionaires: A Social History of Patent Medicines in America before Federal Regulation* (Princeton, N.J.: Princeton University Press, 1961).

5. D. Maurer and V. Vogel, *Narcotics and Narcotic Addiction* (Springfield, Ill.: Charles C. Thomas, 1973).

6. A. Woods, *Dangerous Drugs* (New Haven, Conn.: Yale University Press, 1931).

7. S. Maisto, M. Galizio, and G. Connors, *Drug Use and Misuse* (Fort Worth, Tex.: Harcourt Brace Jovanovich College Publishers, 1991).

8. Young, *The Toadstool Millionaires*, 130–33.

9. J. Furnas, *The Life and Times of the Late Demon Rum* (London: W. H. Allen, 1965). E. Cherrington, ed., *Standard Encyclopedia of the Alcohol*

Problem, 6 vols. (Westerville, Ohio: American Issue Publishing Company, 1925–26). S. Holbrook, *The Golden Age of Quackery* (New York: Macmillan Co., 1959).

10. Young, *The Toadstool Millionaires,* 68.

11. Furnas, *The Life and Times of the Late Demon Rum,* 181.

12. Holbrook, *The Golden Age of Quackery,* 159.

13. S. Lucia, *A History of Wine As Therapy* (Philadelphia: J. B. Lippincott Company, 1963).

14. S. Williams, "The Use of Beverage Alcohol as Medicine, 1790–1860," *Journal of Studies on Alcohol* 41 (1980): 453–66.

15. A. Sinclair, *Era of Excess: A Social History of the Prohibition Movement* (New York: Harper & Row Publishers, 1962).

16. Ibid.

17. American Medical Association, "The Referendum on the Use of Alcohol in the Practice of Medicine," *Journal of the American Medical Association* 74 (7 January 1922): 47–57. A. Wilkerson, "A History of the Concept of Alcoholism as a Disease" (DSW dissertation, University of Pennsylvania, 1966). B. Jones, "A Prohibition Problem: Liquor as Medicine, 1920–1933," *Journal of the History of Medicine and Allied Sciences* 18 (1963): 353–69.

18. B. Fantus, "The Physician and Prohibition," *Journal of the American Medical Association* 74 (24 April 1920): 1144.

19. L. Lewin, *Phantastica: Narcotic and Stimulating Drugs, Their Use and Abuse* (London: Routledge and Kegan Paul, 1931).

20. General references for this section include R. Byck, ed., *Cocaine Papers by Sigmund Freud* (New York: New American Library, 1974) and E. Jones, *The Life and Work of Sigmund Freud* (New York: Basic Books, 1953).

21. D. Musto, "A Study in Cocaine: Sherlock Holmes and Sigmund Freud," *Journal of the American Medical Association* 204, no. 1 (1968): 27–32.

22. Jones, *The Life and Work of Sigmund Freud.*

23. W. Hammond, "Remarks on Cocaine and the So-Called Cocaine Habit," *Journal of Nervous and Mental Disease* 13 (1886): 754–59.

24. J. Spillane, *Modern Drug, Modern Menace: The Legal Use and Distribution of Cocaine in the United States, 1880–1920* (Pittsburgh: Carnegie Mellon University, 1994), 62, 227.

25. W. Bentley, "Erthroxylon Coca in the Opium and Alcohol Habits," *Detroit Therapeutic Gazette* 1 (1880): 253–54.

26. W. White, *Slaying the Dragon: The History of Addiction Treatment and Recovery in America* (Bloomington, Ill.: Chestnut Health Systems, 1998).

27. R. Siegel, "Cocaine and the Privileged Class: A Review of Historical and Contemporary Images," in *Alcohol and Drug Abuse in the Affluent*, ed. B. Stimmel (New York: Haworth Press, 1984).

28. J. Whittaker, "Cocaine for the Opium Habit," *Medical and Surgical Reporter* 53 (1885): 177.

29. M. Pendergrast, *For God, Country and Coca-Cola* (New York: Collier Books, 1993). J. Kennedy, *Coca Exotica: The Illustrated Story of Cocaine* (New York: Cornwwall Books, 1985). L. Gomez, "Cocaine: America's 100 Years of Euphoria and Despair," *Life*, May 1984, 57–67.

30. Spillane, *Modern Drug, Modern Menace*.

31. J. Mattison, "Cocaine Dosage and Cocaine Addiction," *Lancet* (21 May 1887): 1024–25.

32. J. Steele, *Hygienic Physiology with Special Reference to the Use of Alcoholic Drinks and Narcotics* (New York: American Book Company, 1888).

33. T. D. Crothers, *Morphinism and Narcomanias from Other Drugs* (Philadelphia: W. B. Saunders & Company, 1902), 273.

34. T. D. Crothers, "Cocaine Inebriety," *Quarterly Journal of Inebriety* 20 (1898): 369–76.

35. See R. Ashley, *Cocaine: Its History, Uses and Effects* (New York: Warner Books, 1975).

36. General sources for this section include M. Prinzmetal and W. Bloomberg, "The Use of Benzedrine for the Treatment of Narcolepsy," *Journal of the American Medical Association* 105 (1935): 2051. L. Grinspoon and P. Hedblom, *The Speed Culture: Amphetamine Use and Abuse in America* (Cambridge, Mass.: Harvard University Press, 1975). W. L. White and R. Webber, *Cocaine and Other CNS Stimulants* (Bloomington, Ill.: Lighthouse Institute, 1995).

37. Grinspoon and Hedblom, *The Speed Culture*.

38. J. Finlator, *The Drugged Nation* (New York: Simon and Schuster, 1973).

39. W. Armstrong and J. Parascandola, "American Concern over Marijuana in the 1930's," *Pharmacy in History* 14 (1972): 25–34.

40. T. Mikuriya, "Historical Aspects of Cannabis Sativa in Western Medicine," *The New Physician* 18, no. 3 (1969): 902–908. E. Abel, *Marihuana: The First Twelve Thousand Years* (New York: Plenum Press, 1980).

41. Mikuriya, "Historical Aspects of Cannabis Sativa in Western Medicine."

42. P. Tice, *Altered States: Alcohol and Other Drugs in America* (Rochester, N.Y.: Strong Museum, 1992), 52.

43. F. Ludlow, *The Hasheesh Eater* (New York: Harper & Bros, Publishers, 1857).

44. C. Palmer and M. Horowitz, eds., *Shaman Woman, Mainline Lady* (New York: William Morrow, 1982).

45. S. Snyder, "What We Have Forgotten about Pot: A Pharmacologist's History," *New York Times Magazine* (13 December 1970): 26.

46. J. Reichard, "The Marijuana Problem," *Journal of the American Medical Association* 125 (1944): 594–95.

47. Abel, *Marihuana: The First Twelve Thousand Years.*

48. M. Lader, "History of Benzodiazepine Dependence," in *Comprehensive Handbook of Drug and Alcohol Addiction,* ed. N. Miller (New York: Marcel Dekker, Inc., 1991).

49. A. Malcolm, *The Pursuit of Intoxication* (Toronto: Addiction Research Foundation, 1971).

50. J. Etheridge, "Lectures on Chloral Hydrate," *Chicago Medical Journal* 29 (1872): 521–27. Crothers, *Morphinism and Narcomanias from Other Drugs.*

51. H. Kane, *Drugs That Enslave* (1881; reprint, New York: Arno Press, 1981). "Abuse of Chloral Hydrate," *Quarterly Journal of Inebriety* 4 (1880): 53–54.

52. A. Burger, *Drugs and People* (Charlottesville, Va.: University of Virginia Press, 1986).

53. C. Towns, "The Peril of the Drug Habit and the Need for Restrictive Legislation," *Century Magazine* 84 (1912): 580–87.

54. Finlator, *The Drugged Nation.*

55. S. Nuland, *Doctors: The Biography of Medicine* (New York: Vintage Books, 1988).

56. W. Modell, "Mass Drug Catastrophes and the Role of Science and Technology," *Science* 156 (1967): 346–51.

57. B. Stein, *Ludes: A Ballad of the Drug and the Dream* (New York: St. Martin's/Marek, 1982).

58. D. Nagle, "Anesthetic Addiction and Drunkenness: A Contemporary and Historical Review," *International Journal of Addiction* 3 (1968): 23–39.

59. S. Kandall, *Substance and Shadow: Women and Addiction in the United States* (Cambridge, Mass.: Harvard University Press, 1996).

60. B. Grun, *The Timetables of History* (New York: Simon and Schuster, 1979).

61. "The Chloroform Habit As Described by One of Its Victims," *Detroit Lancet* 8 (1884): 251–54.

62. Crothers, *Morphinism and Narcomanias from Other Drugs.*

63. Nuland, *Doctors.*

64. Mikuriya, "Historical Aspects of Cannabis Sativa in Western Medicine," 907.

65. Nagle, "Anesthetic Addiction and Drunkenness," 29.

66. N. Kerr, "Ether Inebriety," *Journal of the American Medical Association* 17 (1891): 791.

67. Lewin, *Phantastica.*

68. Lader, "History of Benzodiazepine Dependence."

69. M. Smith, *Small Comfort: A History of Minor Tranquilizers* (New York: Praeger, 1985).

70. Lader, "History of Benzodiazepine Dependence."

71. W. Mitchell, "The Effects of Anhalonium Lewinii (the Mescal Button)," *British Medical Journal* 2 (1896): 1625. H. Ellis, "A Note on the Phenomena of Mescal Intoxication," *Lancet* 1 (1897): 1540.

72. R. Restak, *Receptors* (New York: Bantam Books, 1994). A. Hofmann, *LSD: My Problem Child* (Los Angeles: Tarcher, 1983).

73. A. Hofmann, "The Discovery of LSD and Subsequent Investigations on Naturally Occurring Hallucinogens," in *Discoveries in Biological Psychiatry,* ed. F. Ayd (Philadelphia: J. B. Lippincott Company, 1970), 91–106.

74. L. Grinspoon and J. Bakalar, "Can Drugs Be Used to Enhance the Psychotherapeutic Process?" *American Journal of Psychotherapy* 40 (July 1986): 393.

75. S. Cohen, *The Substance Abuse Problems: New Issues for the 1980s* (New York: The Haworth Press, 1985).

76. Maurer and Vogel, *Narcotics and Narcotic Addiction.*

77. D. Macht, "The History of Opium and Some of Its Preparations," *Journal of the American Medical Association* 64 (1915): 477–81.

78. D. Musto, "Opium, Cocaine and Marijuana in American History," *Scientific American* (July 1991): 40–47.

79. R. Livingston, ed., *Narcotic Drug Addiction Problems: Proceedings of the Symposium on the History of Narcotic Drug Problems, March 27 and 28, Bethesda, Maryland* (Bethesda, Md.: National Institute of Mental Health, 1959).

80. W. Smith, "An Inaugural Dissertation on Opium Embracing Its History, Chemical Analysis and Use and Abuse As a Medicine," in *Origins of Medical Attitudes Toward Drug Addiction*, ed. G. Grob (1832; reprint, New York: Arno Press, 1981), 21.

81. H. Isbell, "Clinical Research on Addiction in the United States," in *Narcotic Drug Addiction Problems: Proceedings of the Symposium on the History of Narcotic Drug Problems, March 27 and 28, Bethesda, Maryland,* ed. R. Livingston (Bethesda, Md.: National Institute of Mental Health, 1959), 156.

82. D. Courtwright, "Opiate Addiction As a Consequence of the Civil War," *Civil War History* 24 (1978): 101–11. D. Courtwright, "The Hidden Epidemic: Opiate Addiction and Cocaine Use in the South, 1860–1920," *Journal of Southern History* 49 (1983): 57–72.

83. G. Pettey, *Narcotic Drug Diseases and Allied Ailments* (1913; reprint, New York: Arno Press, 1981), 19.

84. R. Schmitz, "Friedrich Wilhelm Sertürner and the Discovery of Morphine," *Pharmacy in History* 27 (1985): 61–74.

85. Crothers, *Morphinism and Narcomanias from Other Drugs.*

86. Macht, "The History of Opium and Some of Its Preparations."

87. C. E. Terry and M. Pellens, *The Opium Problem* (Montclair, N.J.: Patterson Smith, 1928).

88. Quoted in H. Kane, *The Hypodermic Injection of Morphia* (New York: C. L. Birmingham, 1880).

89. R. O'Brien and S. Cohen, *Encyclopedia of Drug Abuse* (Portland, Oreg.: Facts on File, 1992).

90. D. Musto, *The American Disease: Origins of Narcotic Controls* (New Haven, Conn.: Yale University Press, 1973). M. Quinones, "Drug Abuse during the Civil War (1861–1865)," *International Journal of Addiction* 10, no. 6 (1975): 1007–20. Courtwright, "Opiate Addiction As a Consequence of the Civil War."

91. W. Cobbe, *Doctor Judas: A Portrayal of the Opium Habit* (1895; reprint, New York: Arno Press, 1981), 127.

92. D. Musto, "Iatrogenic Addiction: The Problem, Its Definition and History," *Bulletin of the New York Academy of Medicine* 61, 2d series (October 1985): 694–705.

93. Musto, *The American Disease: Origins of Narcotic Controls.* G. Mark, "Racial, Economic and Political Factors in the Development of America's First Drug Laws," *Issues in Criminology* 10, no. 1 (1975): 49–72.

94. Kandall, *Substance and Shadow.*

95. Holbrook, *The Golden Age of Quackery.*

96. T. Pollard, "Use of Opium in Children," *Atlanta Medical and Surgical Journal* 4 (1858): 129–34. J. Haller, "A Short History of the Quack's Materia Medica," *New York State Journal of Medicine* 89 (1989): 520–25.

97. J. Mattison, "Morphinism in the Young," *Atlantic Medical Weekly* 5 (14 March 1896): 165–67.

98. J. Mattison, "Opium Addicts among Medical Men," *Medical Record* 23 (1883): 621–23.

99. T. D. Crothers, "Morphinism among Physicians," *Medical Record* 55 (1899): 784–86.

100. L. Street, *I Was a Drug Addict* (New York: Random House, 1953).

101. P. Lichtenstein, "Narcotic Addiction," *New York Medical Journal* 100 (1914): 962–66.

102. W. White, *The Use and Abuse of Pentazacine (Talwin) in Illinois: A Review with Control Recommendations* (Chicago, Ill.: Illinois Dangerous Drugs Commission, 1978).

103. M. McCormick, *Designer Drug Abuse* (New York: Franklin Watts, 1989). Restak, *Receptors.*

104. McCormick, *Designer Drug Abuse.*

105. J. Shafer, "Designer Drugs," *Science* (March 1985): 66.

106. W. Gallagher, "The Looming Menace of Designer Drugs," *Discover,* August 1986, 24–35.

107. M. Kirsch, *Designer Drugs* (Minneapolis, Minn.: CompCare Publications, 1986).

108. Ibid.

109. Restak, *Receptors,* 115.

110. This discussion is extracted from W. White and R. Webber, "Substance Use Trends: History and Principles," *Counselor* 4, no. 3 (2003): 18–20 and W. White and R. Webber, "The Future of Drug Use in America," *Counselor* 4, no. 4 (2003): 18–20. I would like to acknowledge the assistance of Randal Webber in formulating the principles we believe underlie trends in substance use.

Chapter 5: Addiction As a Family Disease

1. C. Black, *It Will Never Happen to Me* (Denver, Colo.: MAC Publishing, 1981). S. Wegscheider, *Another Chance: Hope and Health for the Alcoholic Family* (Palo Alto, Calif.: Science and Behavior Books, 1981).

2. For further information, see the following two books: S. Brown and V. Lewis, *The Alcoholic Family in Recovery: A Developmental Model* (New York: Guilford Press, 1999) and S. Brown, V. Lewis, and A. Liotta, *The Family Recovery Guide: A Map for Healthy Growth* (Oakland, Calif.: New Harbinger Press, 2000).

ABOUT THE AUTHORS

Drew Pinsky, M.D., is program medical director of chemical dependency services at Las Encinas Hospital in Pasadena, California. He is co-host of the nationally syndicated radio show *Loveline* and the long-running MTV program of the same name. He is author of the best-selling book *Cracked: Putting Broken Lives Together Again.* Dr. Pinsky is well known for his work on *ABC News, Good Morning America,* and CNN. When he is not spending time with his wife, Susan, and their eleven-year-old triplets, he lectures throughout the country and can be seen frequently providing commentary for television talk shows.

Marvin D. Seppala, M.D., is corporate medical director at the Hazelden Foundation. Prior to working at Hazelden, Dr. Seppala was chief of psychiatry and an addiction medicine psychiatric consultant at Springbrook Northwest in Newberg, Oregon. Beginning in the 1980s, Dr. Seppala held a private practice and was a psychiatric consultant to several addiction treatment centers in the Portland, Oregon, and Minneapolis, Minnesota, areas. He is a member of the American Society of Addiction Medicine and a founding member of the Oregon Society of Addiction Medicine. Dr. Seppala is author of *Clinician's Guide to the Twelve Step Principles.* He and his wife, Linda, have two children and live in Wilsonville, Oregon.

Robert J. Meyers, Ph.D., a research associate professor of psychology at the University of New Mexico and associate director of the LifeLink Training Institute in Santa Fe, New Mexico, created the scientifically validated CRAFT model that teaches family members how to intervene on loved ones who are abusing or addicted to alcohol and other drugs. Dr. Meyers is the co-author of *Get Your Loved One Sober: Alternatives to Nagging, Pleading, and Threatening.*

John Gardin, Ph.D., has more than twenty-five years of experience in behavioral health care. He is a licensed psychologist with expertise in the treatment of addictive disorders and sexual abuse. He has also been the medical director and executive director of addiction programs in Oregon and southern California. Currently, Dr. Gardin is a co-founder and co-director of training at the LifeLink Training Institute and director of behavioral health services at the LifeLink family shelter in Santa Fe, New Mexico, and he is an adjunct professor of psychology at the University of New Mexico.

William White, M.A., a senior research consultant at Chestnut Health Systems, has a master's degree in addiction studies and more than thirty-five years of experience working in the addictions field. He has authored/co-authored nine books including *Slaying the Dragon: The History of Addiction Treatment and Recovery in America.*

Stephanie Brown, Ph.D., is a pioneering researcher, clinician, author, teacher, and consultant in the addiction field. She is the director of the Addictions Institute in Menlo Park, California, where she also has a private practice. She is a research associate at the Mental Research Institute in Palo Alto, California, where she co-directs the Family Recovery Research Project. Dr. Brown is the author of eight books. Her most recent book is *A Place Called Self: Women, Sobriety, and Radical Transformation.*

Hazelden Foundation, a national nonprofit organization founded in 1949, helps people reclaim their lives from the disease of addiction. Built on decades of knowledge and experience, Hazelden's comprehensive approach to addiction addresses the full range of individual, family, and professional needs, including addiction treatment and continuing care services for youth and adults, publishing, research, higher learning, public education, and advocacy.

A life of recovery is lived "one day at a time." Hazelden publications, both educational and inspirational, support and strengthen lifelong recovery. In 1954, Hazelden published *Twenty-Four Hours a Day,* the first daily meditation book for recovering alcoholics, and Hazelden continues to publish works to inspire and guide individuals in treatment and recovery, and their loved ones. Professionals who work to prevent and treat addiction also turn to Hazelden for evidence-based curricula, informational materials, and videos for use in schools, treatment programs, and correctional programs.

Through published works, Hazelden extends the reach of hope, encouragement, help, and support to individuals, families, and communities affected by addiction and related issues.

For questions about Hazelden publications, please call **800-328-9000** or visit us online at **hazelden.org/bookstore.**